Anal Addict

Unlocking Extreme Pleasure

Blaze Holeman

ISBN: 9781778905438
Imprint: Telephasic Workshop
Copyright © 2024 Blaze Holeman.
All Rights Reserved.

Contents

Introduction   **1**
The Taboo of Anal Play   1
Understanding the Anatomy   14
Preparing for Anal Play   40
Basic Anal Techniques   66
Advanced Anal Techniques   93
Anal Play in BDSM   129
Exploring Boundaries and Limits   162
Anal Play in Non-Monogamous Relationships   175
Overcoming Challenges and Setbacks   183
Conclusion   194

Index   **209**

Introduction

The Taboo of Anal Play

Overcoming Society's Stigma

The stigma surrounding anal play is deeply rooted in societal norms and cultural perceptions of sexuality. This stigma often manifests as shame, fear, or misunderstanding, which can create barriers to exploring anal pleasure. To overcome these societal stigmas, it is essential to understand their origins, recognize their impact, and actively challenge them.

Understanding the Origins of Stigma

Historically, anal play has been associated with taboo and has often been viewed through a lens of negativity. This stems from various cultural, religious, and social beliefs that frame anal intercourse as deviant or immoral. The perception of anal sex as "dirty" or "shameful" is perpetuated by:

- **Cultural Narratives:** Many cultures have strict norms about sexuality, often promoting heteronormative and penetrative forms of sex while marginalizing alternative practices, including anal play.

- **Religious Doctrine:** Some religious teachings condemn anal sex, leading to internal conflict for individuals who wish to explore this aspect of their sexuality.

- **Media Representation:** The portrayal of anal sex in media often leans towards sensationalism or negativity, reinforcing stereotypes and misconceptions.

Recognizing the Impact of Stigma

The impact of stigma can be profound, leading to feelings of guilt, shame, and isolation for those interested in anal play. This stigma can result in:

- **Fear of Judgment:** Individuals may fear being judged by peers or partners, leading to reluctance in discussing or exploring anal play.

- **Internalized Shame:** The societal narrative can cause individuals to internalize negative beliefs about their desires, leading to shame and self-repression.

- **Limited Communication:** Stigma can hinder open conversations about sexual desires and boundaries, making it difficult to establish trust and intimacy with partners.

Challenging and Overcoming Stigma

To overcome the stigma associated with anal play, it is crucial to engage in a process of education, self-acceptance, and open dialogue. Here are some strategies:

- **Educate Yourself:** Understanding the anatomy and pleasure potential of anal play can empower individuals to embrace their desires. Knowledge dispels myths and fosters a more positive outlook on anal exploration. Consider resources such as sex education books, workshops, and reputable online platforms that provide accurate information.

- **Normalize Conversations:** Create safe spaces for discussing anal play. This can be achieved through open dialogues with partners or friends, participating in sex-positive communities, or attending workshops that focus on sexual exploration. Normalizing these conversations helps dismantle the stigma and fosters understanding.

- **Practice Self-Acceptance:** Embrace your desires without shame. Recognize that sexual preferences are personal and valid. Engaging in self-reflection and affirmations can help combat internalized stigma. One effective technique is to create a positive affirmation statement, such as "My desires are valid, and I deserve pleasure."

- **Seek Support:** If feelings of shame or fear persist, consider seeking support from sex-positive therapists or counselors who can provide guidance and strategies for overcoming stigma. Support groups can also offer a sense of community and shared experience.

- **Advocate for Change:** Engage in conversations about sexual freedom and advocate for a more inclusive understanding of sexuality. Sharing personal experiences and insights can help others recognize the validity of anal play and its potential for pleasure.

Examples of Overcoming Stigma

Numerous individuals have shared their journeys of overcoming the stigma associated with anal play. For instance, a participant in a sex-positive workshop reported how discussing their interests in a supportive environment helped them realize that their desires were not only normal but also widely shared. This realization empowered them to explore anal play with newfound confidence and enthusiasm.

Similarly, a couple who initially faced discomfort discussing anal play found that establishing a safe word and engaging in open dialogue about their boundaries transformed their experiences. They reported that the act of communicating their desires and fears not only enhanced their sexual connection but also deepened their trust in each other.

Conclusion

Overcoming society's stigma surrounding anal play is a journey of education, self-acceptance, and open communication. By understanding the origins of this stigma, recognizing its impact, and actively challenging it, individuals can unlock a world of pleasure and intimacy. Embracing your desires is not just an act of personal empowerment; it is a step towards creating a more open and accepting society where all forms of sexual expression are celebrated.

Breaking Down Barriers

The journey into anal play is often hindered by a myriad of societal, personal, and cultural barriers. To fully embrace this realm of pleasure, it is essential to identify and dismantle these obstacles. This section delves into the various barriers individuals face and offers strategies to overcome them, allowing for a more liberated and fulfilling sexual experience.

Societal Barriers

Society often stigmatizes anal play, associating it with shame, taboo, or even perversion. This stigma can create a significant psychological barrier for individuals interested in exploring anal pleasure. The fear of judgment from peers, family, or society at large can discourage individuals from expressing their desires.

Example: Consider the case of an individual who has always been curious about anal play but refrains from exploring it due to societal norms. They may feel that their interest is abnormal or wrong, leading to internalized shame. This barrier can manifest as anxiety or reluctance to engage in discussions about anal play, even with trusted partners.

Cultural Influences

Cultural beliefs and values play a crucial role in shaping perceptions of sexuality. In many cultures, anal play is viewed as inappropriate or sinful, further entrenching the stigma surrounding it.

Theory: The concept of *cultural relativism* suggests that beliefs and practices should be understood based on the cultural context in which they arise. By applying this theory, individuals can begin to recognize that their cultural background may influence their perceptions of anal play, and that exploring these beliefs can lead to personal growth and acceptance.

Personal Barriers

Beyond societal and cultural influences, personal barriers such as fear, anxiety, and lack of knowledge can impede exploration.

Fear of Pain or Discomfort: Many individuals fear that anal play will be painful or uncomfortable. This fear can stem from a lack of understanding of proper techniques, preparation, and communication with partners.

Example: An individual may have had a negative experience in the past, leading to apprehension about future attempts. This fear can be debilitating, preventing them from enjoying potential pleasure.

Knowledge Gaps

A significant barrier to exploring anal pleasure is the lack of accessible, accurate information. Many individuals rely on myths or misconceptions, which can lead to anxiety and misunderstanding.

Example: The myth that anal play is inherently dirty or unhealthy can deter individuals from exploring this avenue of pleasure. In reality, with proper hygiene and preparation, anal play can be safe and enjoyable.

Strategies for Breaking Down Barriers

To dismantle these barriers, individuals can adopt several strategies:

- **Education:** Seek out reliable sources of information regarding anal play. Books, workshops, and reputable online resources can provide valuable insights into techniques, safety, and the anatomy involved.
- **Open Communication:** Engage in honest conversations with partners about desires, fears, and boundaries. Establishing a safe space for dialogue can alleviate anxiety and foster trust.
- **Gradual Exploration:** Start with small steps. Begin by exploring external anal stimulation before progressing to internal play. This gradual approach can help build confidence and reduce fear.
- **Community Support:** Connect with communities or groups that celebrate sexual exploration. Sharing experiences and learning from others can provide encouragement and reduce feelings of isolation.
- **Therapeutic Support:** For individuals struggling with deeply rooted fears or anxieties, seeking the help of a therapist specializing in sexual health can be beneficial. Therapy can provide tools to navigate personal barriers and enhance overall sexual well-being.

Conclusion

Breaking down the barriers to anal play is a vital step toward embracing one's sexual desires. By addressing societal stigma, cultural influences, personal fears, and knowledge gaps, individuals can create a more open and accepting relationship with their sexuality. The journey may require patience and persistence, but the rewards of exploration, connection, and pleasure are well worth the effort. Embrace the challenge of dismantling these barriers, and unlock the potential for profound pleasure and intimacy.

Embracing Your Desires

Embracing your desires is an essential step in the journey of sexual exploration, particularly when it comes to anal play. This section aims to empower you to accept and celebrate your desires without shame or fear. Understanding the importance of embracing your desires can lead to more fulfilling sexual experiences and deeper connections with yourself and your partners.

Understanding Desire

Desire is a natural and intrinsic part of human sexuality. It encompasses a wide range of feelings, from curiosity to longing, and can manifest in various ways. According to the *Kinsey Reports*, sexual desire varies significantly among individuals and is influenced by numerous factors, including biological, psychological, and social aspects. Embracing your desires means acknowledging and validating them, regardless of societal norms or personal insecurities.

The Role of Societal Norms

Societal norms often dictate what is considered acceptable in sexual expression. Anal play, in particular, has historically been surrounded by stigma and misconceptions. Many people may feel ashamed or guilty about their interest in anal play due to cultural taboos. It's crucial to recognize that these societal constructs do not define your worth or the validity of your desires.

To illustrate, consider the following scenario: A person might feel an intense desire to explore anal sex but hesitate due to fear of judgment or rejection. By confronting these societal norms and reframing their understanding of desire, they can begin to embrace their interest as a natural part of their sexuality.

The Importance of Self-Acceptance

Self-acceptance is a vital component of embracing your desires. It involves recognizing that your sexual preferences are valid and worthy of exploration. Engaging in self-reflection can help you understand your desires better. Ask yourself questions such as:

- What excites me about anal play?
- What fears or insecurities do I have regarding my desires?
- How can I communicate my desires to my partner(s)?

By taking the time to explore these questions, you can foster a deeper connection with your desires and enhance your sexual experiences.

Communication with Partners

Once you have embraced your desires, the next step is to communicate them effectively with your partner(s). Open dialogue about sexual preferences can strengthen intimacy and trust in a relationship. Here are some tips for discussing your desires:

1. **Choose the Right Time and Place:** Find a comfortable and private setting to discuss your desires without distractions.
2. **Be Honest and Direct:** Clearly express what you want to explore and why it excites you.
3. **Encourage Openness:** Invite your partner to share their desires and concerns, creating a safe space for mutual exploration.

For example, you might say, "I've been thinking about trying anal play. I find the idea exciting, and I'd love to explore it with you if you're open to it." This approach fosters a collaborative atmosphere where both partners can express their interests and boundaries.

Addressing Fears and Insecurities

It's normal to have fears and insecurities when it comes to exploring new sexual territories. Common concerns about anal play include pain, loss of control, and feelings of vulnerability. To address these fears, consider the following strategies:

- **Educate Yourself:** Knowledge is power. Understanding the anatomy involved, safety precautions, and techniques can alleviate fears about pain or discomfort.
- **Start Slow:** Gradual exploration can help build confidence. Begin with external stimulation or smaller toys before progressing to penetration.

- **Practice Mindfulness:** Techniques such as deep breathing and visualization can help manage anxiety. Focus on the sensations and pleasure rather than the fear.

Celebrating Your Desires

Once you've embraced and communicated your desires, it's essential to celebrate them. Engaging in activities that affirm your sexuality can enhance your overall sexual experience. This can include:

- **Self-Exploration:** Take time to explore your body and discover what feels pleasurable. This can help you understand your desires better and build confidence.

- **Creating a Safe Space:** Design a comfortable environment for sexual exploration, free from distractions or judgment.

- **Engaging with Communities:** Connecting with like-minded individuals or communities can provide support and validation for your desires.

For instance, participating in workshops or discussions about anal play can foster a sense of belonging and encourage you to embrace your desires more fully.

Conclusion

Embracing your desires is a powerful act of self-acceptance and empowerment. By confronting societal norms, communicating openly with partners, addressing fears, and celebrating your interests, you can unlock new dimensions of pleasure and intimacy. Remember, your desires are valid, and exploring them can lead to profound personal growth and satisfaction. Embrace the journey of discovery, and allow yourself the freedom to experience the pleasure that awaits.

Importance of Consent and Communication

In the realm of anal play, the concepts of consent and communication are paramount. Engaging in any form of sexual activity requires a mutual agreement between all parties involved, ensuring that everyone feels safe, respected, and enthusiastic about their choices. This section will explore the critical importance of consent and communication, the theoretical frameworks that support these principles, common challenges, and practical examples to foster healthy sexual experiences.

Theoretical Frameworks of Consent

Consent is not merely a checkbox to be ticked; it is an ongoing dialogue that evolves with each interaction. According to the **Enthusiastic Consent Model**, consent must be given freely, actively, and without coercion. This model emphasizes that consent should be enthusiastic, meaning that all parties should express a genuine desire to participate in the activity.

$$C = E + F + A \qquad (1)$$

Where:

- C = Consent
- E = Enthusiasm
- F = Freedom from coercion
- A = Active participation

This equation illustrates that consent is a composite of enthusiasm, freedom from coercion, and active involvement. Each component is essential for a healthy sexual experience, particularly in anal play, where trust and comfort are vital.

Communication: The Cornerstone of Consent

Effective communication is the cornerstone of ensuring consent is informed and ongoing. It involves discussing desires, boundaries, and any potential concerns before engaging in anal play. Open dialogue fosters a sense of safety and trust, allowing partners to express their feelings and preferences freely.

- **Establishing Safe Words:** Safe words are predetermined signals that indicate when a partner feels uncomfortable or wishes to stop. For example, using a color code (e.g., "red" for stop, "yellow" for slow down) can facilitate clear communication during play.
- **Checking In:** Regularly checking in with your partner during anal play is crucial. Phrases such as "How are you feeling?" or "Is this okay?" can encourage partners to share their experiences and adjust accordingly.
- **Post-Play Debriefing:** Aftercare and debriefing allow partners to discuss their experiences, feelings, and any discomfort they might have felt during the activity. This practice not only enhances intimacy but also reinforces trust for future encounters.

Challenges in Consent and Communication

Despite the importance of consent and communication, several challenges can arise:

- **Societal Stigma:** The stigma surrounding anal play can lead to feelings of shame or embarrassment, making it difficult for individuals to express their desires or boundaries. Overcoming societal norms requires conscious effort and support from partners.

- **Fear of Rejection:** Individuals may fear that expressing their desires could lead to rejection or judgment from their partner. This fear can stifle open communication and hinder the establishment of consent.

- **Misinterpretation:** Non-verbal cues can sometimes be misinterpreted. It is essential to clarify intentions and feelings verbally to avoid misunderstandings that could lead to discomfort or harm.

Practical Examples of Consent and Communication

To illustrate the importance of consent and communication in anal play, consider the following scenarios:

- **Scenario 1: The Initial Conversation**

    "Hey, I've been thinking about exploring anal play together. How do you feel about that?"

This question opens the door for discussion, allowing both partners to express their thoughts and feelings without pressure.

- **Scenario 2: Establishing Boundaries**

    "I'm interested in trying anal, but I want to set some boundaries first. I'm not comfortable with anything too intense right away."

This statement clearly communicates limits, ensuring that both partners understand each other's comfort levels.

- **Scenario 3: Using Safe Words**

    "If at any point you feel uncomfortable, just say 'red' and we'll stop immediately."

This establishes a safety net, allowing partners to engage in anal play with the assurance that they can halt the activity at any time.

- **Scenario 4: Post-Play Check-In**

    "How did you feel about our experience? Is there anything you'd like to do differently next time?"

    This fosters a culture of continuous improvement in communication and consent, enhancing future encounters.

Conclusion

In conclusion, the importance of consent and communication in anal play cannot be overstated. By understanding the theoretical frameworks that underpin these principles, addressing common challenges, and employing practical strategies for effective dialogue, individuals can create a safe and pleasurable environment for exploration. Remember, consent is an ongoing process, and open communication is the key to unlocking the full potential of your anal journey. Embrace the empowering nature of consent, and let it guide your exploration into the depths of pleasure.

Safety Precautions

Engaging in anal play can be an incredibly pleasurable experience, but it is crucial to prioritize safety to ensure that everyone involved has a positive and enjoyable time. This section will discuss essential safety precautions that should be taken before, during, and after anal play to minimize risks and enhance the overall experience.

Understanding Risks

Before diving into the specifics of safety precautions, it is important to understand the potential risks associated with anal play. These risks may include:

- **Injury:** The anal area is sensitive and can be prone to tears or other injuries if not approached with care.

- **Infections:** The rectum contains bacteria that can lead to infections if proper hygiene is not observed.

- **Transmission of STIs:** Anal intercourse can increase the risk of sexually transmitted infections (STIs) if protective measures are not taken.

By being aware of these risks, you can take proactive steps to mitigate them.

Pre-Play Preparations

Hygiene Practices   Maintaining hygiene is vital for safe anal play. Here are some recommended practices:

- **Cleansing:** Before engaging in anal play, it is advisable to clean the anal area thoroughly. This can be done with warm water and mild soap. Some individuals may choose to use an enema for internal cleansing, but this should be done cautiously and not excessively, as it can disrupt the natural flora of the rectum.

- **Nail Care:** Ensure that fingernails are trimmed and smooth to avoid any accidental scratches or tears during anal play.

- **Toy Cleaning:** If using toys, ensure they are cleaned properly before and after use. Use a suitable cleaner or soap and water, and consider using a dedicated toy cleaner for added safety.

Lubrication Techniques   Proper lubrication is essential for a pleasurable and safe experience. The anus does not produce natural lubrication, so it is important to use a high-quality lubricant. Here are some tips:

- **Choose the Right Lubricant:** Water-based lubricants are easy to clean but may require reapplication. Silicone-based lubricants last longer and are great for anal play but should not be used with silicone toys. Oil-based lubricants can provide a smooth experience but may not be safe with latex condoms.

- **Apply Generously:** Apply lubricant generously to both the anal area and any toys or fingers being used. Reapply as necessary to maintain comfort and reduce friction.

During Play: Communication and Consent

Establishing Boundaries   Communication is key to a safe and enjoyable experience. Before engaging in anal play, have an open discussion with your partner(s) about desires, boundaries, and limits. This includes:

- **Discussing Comfort Levels:** Talk about what each person is comfortable with, including any specific activities or techniques that may be off-limits.

- **Setting Safe Words:** Establish a safe word or signal that anyone can use if they feel uncomfortable or need to stop. This allows for immediate communication during play.

Listening to Your Body During anal play, it is essential to pay attention to your body and your partner's reactions. If any pain or discomfort arises, stop immediately and assess the situation. Remember that pleasure should always be the primary goal.

Post-Play Considerations

Aftercare Aftercare is an important aspect of any intimate experience, especially after anal play. It involves taking time to reconnect and care for each other following the session. This can include:

- **Physical Comfort:** Cuddle, talk, or provide any physical comfort that may be needed.

- **Hygiene:** After anal play, it is important to clean the anal area again to prevent infections. This includes washing hands and any toys used.

- **Emotional Check-In:** Discuss the experience with your partner(s) to address any feelings or concerns that may have arisen during play. This helps in building trust and improving future experiences.

Monitoring for Complications After anal play, be aware of any unusual symptoms such as bleeding, severe pain, or signs of infection (e.g., fever, unusual discharge). If any of these occur, seek medical attention promptly.

Conclusion

In conclusion, safety precautions are paramount when engaging in anal play. By understanding the risks, preparing adequately, communicating openly, and practicing proper hygiene, you can create a safe and pleasurable environment for exploration. Remember, anal play is about mutual enjoyment and trust; prioritize safety to ensure that both you and your partner(s) can fully embrace the experience. Embrace your desires, and let safety guide your journey into the world of anal pleasure.

Understanding the Anatomy

Female Anal Anatomy

Understanding female anal anatomy is crucial for anyone looking to explore anal play safely and pleasurably. The anatomy of the anal region is complex, involving not only the external structures but also the internal anatomy that plays a significant role in sexual pleasure. This section will break down the anatomy of the female anal region, focusing on key structures, their functions, and how they contribute to pleasure.

External Structures

The external anal area, often referred to as the perineum, is the region between the vagina and the anus. This area is rich in nerve endings, making it highly sensitive to touch. The key external structures include:

- **Anus:** The anus is the opening at the end of the digestive tract. It is surrounded by the anal sphincter, a ring of muscle that controls the passage of stool and gas. The anal sphincter consists of two parts: the internal anal sphincter, which is involuntary, and the external anal sphincter, which is under voluntary control.

- **Perineum:** The perineum is the area of skin that stretches from the vaginal opening to the anus. This area can be stimulated during anal play, enhancing pleasure.

- **Labia:** The labia majora and labia minora are the outer and inner folds of skin surrounding the vaginal opening. While not directly part of the anal anatomy, they can be involved in anal play, as they are sensitive to touch and can enhance arousal.

Internal Structures

Internally, the anatomy of the female anal region is just as important. The internal structures include:

- **Rectum:** The rectum is the final section of the large intestine, leading from the sigmoid colon to the anus. It is about 12 cm long and can expand to accommodate the passage of stool or other objects during anal play. The rectal walls are elastic and can provide pleasurable sensations when stimulated.

UNDERSTANDING THE ANATOMY

- **Anal Canal:** The anal canal is the passage leading from the rectum to the anus, measuring approximately 2.5 to 4 cm in length. The lining of the anal canal is sensitive and contains a high density of nerve endings, making it particularly responsive to stimulation.
- **Pelvic Floor Muscles:** The pelvic floor muscles support the pelvic organs and play a crucial role in sexual function. Strengthening these muscles can enhance anal pleasure and improve control during anal play.

The Role of the G-spot

While the G-spot is primarily associated with vaginal stimulation, it can also be influenced by anal play. The G-spot is located on the anterior wall of the vagina, about 2.5 to 7.5 cm inside. When anal penetration occurs, especially during deep thrusting, the G-spot can be indirectly stimulated, leading to heightened pleasure.

Techniques for Stimulating the G-spot

When engaging in anal play, consider the following techniques to enhance G-spot stimulation:

- **Angled Penetration:** Positioning the penetrating object (fingers, toys, or penis) at an angle can help target the G-spot while simultaneously stimulating the anal area.
- **Rhythmic Thrusting:** Alternating between deep and shallow thrusts can create a pleasurable rhythm that stimulates both the G-spot and the anal region.
- **Use of Toys:** Utilizing toys designed for dual stimulation can effectively target both the G-spot and the anal area simultaneously. Look for toys that have a curved design or a dual-ended structure.

The Connection between Anal and Vaginal Pleasure

The connection between anal and vaginal pleasure is rooted in the shared nerve pathways and anatomical proximity. Engaging in anal play can heighten sensitivity in the vaginal area, leading to more intense orgasms. The interplay of sensations can create a unique and pleasurable experience that enhances overall sexual satisfaction.

Conclusion

Understanding female anal anatomy is essential for safe and pleasurable anal play. By familiarizing oneself with the external and internal structures, as well as the connections to other forms of sexual pleasure, individuals can explore their desires with confidence. Embracing this knowledge not only enhances personal experiences but also fosters a deeper connection with one's body and sexuality.

$$P = \frac{F}{A} \qquad (2)$$

Where P is the pressure applied during anal play, F is the force exerted, and A is the area over which the force is applied. This equation can remind practitioners to be mindful of the pressure they apply during anal play to ensure comfort and pleasure.

In summary, the exploration of female anal anatomy opens the door to new realms of pleasure. By understanding the intricacies of the body, individuals can unlock new experiences and embrace their desires fully.

External and Internal Structures

Anal anatomy is fascinating and complex, encompassing a variety of external and internal structures that play crucial roles in pleasure and function. Understanding these structures is essential for anyone looking to explore anal play safely and enjoyably.

External Structures

The external anal structures include the anus itself, which is the opening at the end of the digestive tract, and the surrounding tissues. The key components of the external anatomy are:

- **Anus:** The anus is a muscular opening that allows for the expulsion of waste. It is surrounded by the anal sphincters, which are crucial for maintaining control over bowel movements and, importantly, for anal play.

- **Anal Sphincters:** There are two main sphincters: the internal anal sphincter, which is involuntary and helps maintain closure, and the external anal sphincter, which is voluntary and allows for conscious control. Understanding how to relax these muscles is essential for enjoyable anal play.

- **Perineum:** This is the area between the anus and the genitals. It is rich in nerve endings and can be a source of significant pleasure when stimulated.
- **Gluteal Muscles:** The muscles of the buttocks also play a role in anal play, as they can enhance sensations during penetration and can be engaged or relaxed to control the experience.

Internal Structures

The internal anal structures extend beyond the anus into the rectum and beyond. Here are the key components:

- **Rectum:** The rectum is the final section of the large intestine, approximately 12 to 15 centimeters long. It serves as a temporary storage site for feces before elimination. During anal play, the rectum can accommodate various objects, including fingers and toys, but it's vital to ensure that any insertion is done gently and with adequate lubrication.
- **Anal Canal:** The anal canal is the short passage leading from the rectum to the anus, typically about 2.5 to 4 centimeters in length. This area is highly sensitive and contains many nerve endings, making it a focal point for pleasure during anal stimulation.
- **Nerve Endings:** The anal region is densely packed with nerve endings, particularly in the anal canal and sphincters. Stimulation of these areas can result in intense pleasure, and understanding how to stimulate these nerves can enhance the experience.
- **Prostate Gland (in Males):** Located about 5 to 7 centimeters inside the rectum, the prostate gland can be stimulated through the rectal wall. This gland is often referred to as the male G-spot and can produce intense pleasure when massaged. Techniques for prostate stimulation vary but often include a combination of pressure and rhythmic movement.

The Importance of Understanding These Structures

Understanding the external and internal structures of the anal region is crucial for a variety of reasons:

- **Safety:** Knowledge of anatomy helps prevent injury during anal play. For instance, knowing the location of the anal sphincters and the rectum can guide gentle and respectful exploration.

- **Enhancing Pleasure:** Familiarity with the sensitive areas can lead to more pleasurable experiences. For example, stimulating the perineum while engaging in anal play can heighten sensations.
- **Communication:** Understanding these structures allows for better communication with partners about what feels good and what doesn't. This can lead to a more fulfilling and enjoyable experience for all parties involved.

Common Problems and Considerations

While exploring anal play, individuals may encounter challenges. Here are some common issues and considerations:

- **Discomfort or Pain:** It is essential to differentiate between pleasure and pain. If discomfort occurs, it may indicate that more lubrication is needed, or that the pace should be slowed down. Communication with partners is vital to address any discomfort immediately.
- **Hygiene:** Maintaining cleanliness is crucial for anal play. Proper hygiene practices, such as washing hands and toys before and after use, can prevent infections and promote a safe experience.
- **Relaxation Techniques:** Many individuals may feel tense or anxious about anal play. Techniques such as deep breathing, warm baths, or gentle massages can help relax the body and facilitate a more enjoyable experience.

Conclusion

By understanding the external and internal structures of the anal region, individuals can approach anal play with confidence and knowledge. This understanding not only enhances pleasure but also promotes safety and communication, making the journey into anal exploration both fulfilling and enjoyable. As you continue to explore, remember that every body is different, and what works for one person may not work for another. Embrace the journey of discovery and enjoy the myriad of sensations that anal play can offer.

The Role of the G-spot

The G-spot, often referred to as the Grafenberg spot, is a highly debated and intriguing area located within the vaginal canal, typically a few inches in from the vaginal opening, on the anterior wall (the side closest to the abdomen). While

UNDERSTANDING THE ANATOMY

some individuals report intense pleasure when this area is stimulated, others may not experience the same sensations. Understanding the G-spot's role in anal play can enhance sexual experiences for both partners and unlock new realms of pleasure.

Anatomy of the G-spot

The G-spot is thought to be an extension of the clitoral network, consisting of erectile tissue that engorges when aroused. This area is rich in nerve endings and is believed to be closely linked to the urethra, which may explain the sensations of fullness or urgency some individuals experience during stimulation. The G-spot can vary in size and sensitivity from person to person, and its location can also shift due to factors such as arousal and individual anatomy.

The Connection Between the G-spot and Anal Play

The G-spot's proximity to the anus creates a unique opportunity for simultaneous stimulation during anal play. Many individuals find that when the G-spot is stimulated, it can heighten the sensations experienced during anal penetration, leading to a more intense overall experience. This connection can be explored through various techniques, such as:

- **Fingering Techniques:** Using one or two fingers to apply pressure on the G-spot while simultaneously stimulating the anus can create a pleasurable feedback loop.

- **Toy Play:** Anal toys designed to target both the G-spot and the anal area can provide dual stimulation, enhancing pleasure.

- **Partner Techniques:** In a partnered setting, one partner can focus on anal penetration while the other stimulates the G-spot, creating a harmonious experience.

Techniques for Stimulating the G-spot

To effectively stimulate the G-spot, consider the following techniques:

1. **Curved Finger Technique:** Insert one or two fingers into the vagina and curl them upwards towards the belly button. Apply firm, rhythmic pressure to the G-spot area.

2. **Pressure and Release:** Experiment with varying pressure levels. Some individuals may prefer a gentle touch, while others enjoy firmer pressure.

3. **Vibrators:** Use a vibrator designed for internal use, ensuring it has a curve or angle to effectively target the G-spot.

4. **Combination Play:** Simultaneously stimulate the G-spot while engaging in anal play, either through fingers or toys, to amplify sensations.

Common Problems and Misconceptions

Despite its reputation, the G-spot is not universally pleasurable for everyone. Some common issues include:

- **Sensitivity Variability:** Not all individuals experience pleasure from G-spot stimulation. Factors such as arousal levels, comfort, and personal anatomy can influence sensitivity.

- **Pain vs. Pleasure:** Some may confuse discomfort with pleasure, particularly if they are new to anal or G-spot stimulation. It is crucial to communicate openly and ensure that both partners feel comfortable.

- **The Myth of the G-spot:** Some argue that the G-spot does not exist or is merely a psychological construct. However, many report pleasurable sensations from G-spot stimulation, indicating that individual experiences may vary widely.

Examples of G-spot Stimulation in Anal Play

Here are a few scenarios that illustrate the role of the G-spot in anal play:

- **Solo Exploration:** An individual may use a curved dildo designed for dual stimulation, inserting it anally while simultaneously applying pressure to the G-spot, allowing for a unique exploration of pleasure.

- **Partner Play:** During intercourse, a partner may focus on anal penetration while the receiving partner uses their fingers or a toy to stimulate their G-spot, creating layers of sensation.

- **Experimentation with Angles:** Adjusting the angle of penetration can enhance G-spot stimulation. For example, when in a doggy-style position, the angle may naturally stimulate the G-spot while allowing for anal play.

UNDERSTANDING THE ANATOMY

Conclusion

The G-spot plays a significant role in enhancing pleasure during anal play, providing opportunities for deeper connections and heightened sensations. Understanding its anatomy, exploring various techniques, and communicating openly with partners can lead to fulfilling and pleasurable experiences. As with all aspects of sexual exploration, patience, consent, and a willingness to experiment are key to unlocking the full potential of anal and G-spot pleasure.

$$\text{Pleasure} = \text{G-spot Stimulation} + \text{Anal Stimulation} \tag{3}$$

By embracing the G-spot's role in anal play, individuals can embark on a journey of discovery and empowerment, celebrating their bodies and desires.

Techniques for Stimulating the G-spot

The G-spot, often referred to as the Grafenberg spot, is an erogenous zone located on the anterior (front) wall of the vagina, approximately 1 to 3 inches inside. It is believed to be a sensitive area that, when stimulated, can lead to heightened sexual arousal and even orgasm for some individuals. In this section, we will explore various techniques for effectively stimulating the G-spot, addressing potential challenges, and providing practical examples to enhance pleasure.

Understanding the G-spot

The G-spot is not a distinct anatomical structure but rather a region that may contain a cluster of sensitive nerve endings, erectile tissue, and glands. When stimulated, this area can swell and become more pronounced, which may enhance pleasure. The experience of G-spot stimulation varies from person to person; some may find it intensely pleasurable, while others may not experience significant sensations.

Preparation for G-spot Stimulation

Before diving into G-spot stimulation techniques, it is essential to ensure that both partners are comfortable and relaxed. Here are some preparatory steps:

- **Communication:** Discuss desires, boundaries, and any concerns about G-spot stimulation. Establishing a safe word can enhance comfort and trust.
- **Hygiene:** Ensure cleanliness by washing hands and any toys that will be used. This not only promotes safety but also adds to the overall experience.

- **Arousal:** Engage in foreplay to increase arousal. This can include kissing, oral sex, and other forms of stimulation to prepare the body for G-spot exploration.

Basic Techniques for G-spot Stimulation

Once both partners are ready, the following techniques can be employed to stimulate the G-spot effectively:

1. **Fingering Technique:**

    - **Positioning:** Have the receiving partner lie on their back with their knees bent or in a comfortable position that allows access to the vagina.
    - **Insertion:** Insert one or two fingers into the vagina, curling them in a "come hither" motion towards the front wall. The G-spot is typically located about 1 to 3 inches in, so gentle pressure should be applied.
    - **Rhythm:** Experiment with different rhythms and pressures. Some may prefer a steady motion, while others may enjoy varying the intensity.

2. **Using a Toy:**

    - **Choosing the Right Toy:** Select a G-spot vibrator or a curved dildo designed for G-spot stimulation. These toys often feature a shape that allows for targeted pressure.
    - **Technique:** Insert the toy into the vagina and angle it towards the front wall. Use a rocking or thrusting motion to stimulate the G-spot directly.

3. **Partner Positioning:**

    - **Missionary Position:** In this classic position, the receiving partner lies on their back while the penetrating partner enters. The penetrating partner can angle their thrusts to apply pressure to the G-spot.
    - **Doggy Style:** This position allows for deeper penetration and can create a natural angle for G-spot stimulation. The penetrating partner can adjust their thrusting angle to target the G-spot effectively.

Advanced Techniques for G-spot Stimulation

Once basic techniques are mastered, consider exploring advanced methods for deeper pleasure:

1. **Combination Stimulation:**
    + Combining clitoral stimulation with G-spot stimulation can enhance arousal and lead to more intense orgasms. This can be achieved through simultaneous finger or toy stimulation on both the G-spot and clitoris.

2. **Pressure Play:**
    + Experiment with varying degrees of pressure on the G-spot. Some individuals may enjoy firm pressure, while others may prefer gentler touches. Use your partner's feedback to guide your actions.

3. **Thrusting Techniques:**
    + When using a toy or during penetration, try varying the thrusting techniques. Slow, deep thrusts may provide a different sensation compared to quick, shallow thrusts. Pay attention to your partner's reactions to find what feels best.

Addressing Challenges

While G-spot stimulation can be pleasurable, it may also present challenges. Here are some common issues and solutions:

- **Difficulty Locating the G-spot:** If locating the G-spot proves challenging, encourage exploration. Different positions or angles may reveal the sensitive area more effectively.
- **Discomfort or Pain:** If discomfort arises, stop and reassess. Ensure adequate lubrication and relaxation. Communicating openly about sensations can help address any issues.
- **Emotional Responses:** G-spot stimulation can elicit strong emotional reactions. Be prepared for feelings of vulnerability or unexpected emotions and approach them with care and compassion.

Conclusion

Stimulating the G-spot can open new avenues of pleasure and exploration for individuals and couples alike. By understanding the anatomy, employing various techniques, and communicating openly, partners can create a fulfilling experience that embraces the joys of G-spot stimulation. Remember, every body is unique, and what works for one person may not work for another. Embrace the journey of discovery and enjoy the pleasures that come with it.

The Connection between Anal and Vaginal Pleasure

Anal and vaginal pleasure are often viewed as distinct experiences; however, they are intricately connected through anatomy, physiological responses, and shared nerve pathways. Understanding this connection can enhance sexual experiences and broaden the spectrum of pleasure for individuals and their partners.

Anatomical Overlap

The human body is a remarkable system where different parts work in harmony. The anus and vagina are in close proximity, separated by the perineum, which is a highly sensitive area. This proximity means that stimulation in one area can lead to heightened sensations in the other.

$$\text{Pleasure} = f(\text{Stimulation}_{\text{anal}}) + f(\text{Stimulation}_{\text{vaginal}}) \qquad (4)$$

This equation suggests that the overall pleasure experienced can be a function of both anal and vaginal stimulation. When one area is stimulated, it can increase blood flow and sensitivity in the other area due to the shared nerve supply.

Nerve Pathways and Sensation

The pudendal nerve, which is the primary nerve responsible for sensation in the genital region, serves both the anus and the vagina. Stimulation of the anal area can lead to increased sensitivity in the vaginal area, and vice versa. This phenomenon can be explained through the concept of referred sensation, where stimulation of one area creates sensations in another.

Physiological Responses

Both anal and vaginal stimulation can trigger similar physiological responses, including increased heart rate, heightened arousal, and the release of endorphins. The body's response to pleasure is a complex interplay of various systems, including the nervous and hormonal systems.

$$\text{Arousal} = \text{Endorphins} + \text{Blood Flow} + \text{Nerve Stimulation} \qquad (5)$$

As arousal increases through either anal or vaginal stimulation, the body becomes more responsive to further stimulation in both areas, creating a cycle of pleasure that can be amplified through techniques that engage both.

Techniques for Combining Pleasure

To fully explore the connection between anal and vaginal pleasure, individuals can employ several techniques:

- **Simultaneous Stimulation:** Engaging in anal and vaginal stimulation at the same time can create a profound sense of pleasure. For instance, using fingers or toys to stimulate both areas can enhance the overall experience.
- **Alternating Focus:** Switching focus between anal and vaginal stimulation during sexual activity can create an ebb and flow of sensations that keeps the experience fresh and exciting.
- **Using Lubrication:** Ensuring adequate lubrication is essential for both anal and vaginal play. This reduces friction and enhances pleasure, allowing for smoother transitions between the two forms of stimulation.

Psychological Aspects

The psychological connection between anal and vaginal pleasure is equally important. Many individuals report that engaging in anal play can enhance their overall sexual experience, leading to a deeper sense of intimacy and connection with their partner.

$$\text{Intimacy} = \text{Trust} + \text{Communication} + \text{Shared Experience} \qquad (6)$$

When partners communicate openly about their desires and boundaries, they can create a safe space to explore anal and vaginal pleasure together. This shared journey can foster greater intimacy and trust, making the experience more fulfilling.

Common Challenges

Despite the potential for enhanced pleasure, some individuals may face challenges when exploring the connection between anal and vaginal play. These can include:

- **Fear of Pain:** Concerns about discomfort can inhibit exploration. It's important to approach anal play with patience and to use proper techniques, such as relaxation and adequate lubrication.

- **Societal Stigma:** Cultural attitudes toward anal play can create feelings of shame or embarrassment. Overcoming these societal barriers through education and open discussion can empower individuals to embrace their desires.

- **Physical Limitations:** Some individuals may have physical limitations that make certain activities challenging. Adaptations and modifications can be made to accommodate different bodies and preferences.

Conclusion

The connection between anal and vaginal pleasure is a testament to the body's intricate design and the potential for pleasure that lies within. By understanding the anatomical, physiological, and psychological connections, individuals can enrich their sexual experiences and explore new realms of pleasure. Embracing this connection not only enhances personal satisfaction but also fosters deeper intimacy and communication between partners.

In summary, the interplay of anal and vaginal pleasure is not only about physical sensations but also about emotional connections and shared experiences. Whether through simultaneous stimulation, alternating focus, or simply exploring the boundaries of pleasure, the journey can lead to profound discoveries about oneself and one's partner.

Male Anal Anatomy

Understanding male anal anatomy is essential for anyone exploring anal play. The male anatomy includes various external and internal structures that contribute to pleasure. This section will delve into these anatomical features, their functions, and how they can enhance sexual experiences.

External Structures

The external structures of male anal anatomy consist of the anus and surrounding areas. The anus is the opening at the end of the digestive tract and is surrounded by the anal sphincter muscles, which control the expulsion of feces. The sphincters consist of two main parts:

- **Internal Anal Sphincter:** This is an involuntary muscle that helps maintain continence. It is controlled by the autonomic nervous system and remains contracted at rest.

- **External Anal Sphincter:** This is a voluntary muscle that allows for conscious control over the anal opening. It can be contracted or relaxed at will, making it essential for anal play.

The perineum, the area between the anus and the scrotum, is also an important part of male anatomy. It is highly sensitive and can be stimulated to enhance pleasure during anal activities.

Internal Structures

Internally, the male anal anatomy includes several key components that contribute to sexual pleasure:

- **Rectum:** The rectum is the last section of the large intestine, leading from the sigmoid colon to the anus. It is approximately 15 to 20 centimeters long and can accommodate various objects, making it a significant area for anal stimulation.
- **Prostate Gland:** Located about 5 to 7 centimeters inside the rectum, the prostate is often referred to as the male G-spot. It is walnut-sized and can be stimulated through the rectal wall. The prostate plays a crucial role in sexual pleasure and ejaculation. Stimulation of this gland can produce intense orgasms and even prostate orgasms, which are distinct from traditional orgasms.
- **Seminal Vesicles and Vas Deferens:** These structures are involved in the production and transport of semen. While they are not directly involved in anal play, understanding their location can enhance awareness of the male reproductive system.

The Role of the Prostate in Pleasure

The prostate gland is a critical component of male anal anatomy. Its stimulation can lead to heightened sexual arousal and orgasm. The prostate is sensitive to pressure and can be stimulated in various ways:

- **Direct Stimulation:** This can be achieved through fingers or toys inserted into the rectum, applying pressure to the prostate.
- **Indirect Stimulation:** Techniques such as perineal massage can also provide pleasurable sensations by stimulating the area surrounding the prostate.

Techniques for Prostate Stimulation

To effectively stimulate the prostate, consider the following techniques:

1. **Fingers:** Insert one or two fingers into the rectum, curling them forward towards the belly button to locate the prostate. Apply gentle pressure and explore different rhythms and intensities.

2. **Toys:** There are specially designed prostate massagers that can provide targeted stimulation. Choose toys with a flared base for safety and comfort.

3. **Vibrators:** Using a vibrating toy can enhance the sensations experienced during prostate stimulation, leading to more intense orgasms.

It is essential to communicate with your partner about preferences and comfort levels during prostate play.

Combining Prostate Stimulation with Other Forms of Pleasure

Prostate stimulation can be combined with other forms of sexual pleasure for a more fulfilling experience. Here are a few suggestions:

- **Simultaneous Stimulation:** Combining prostate stimulation with penile stimulation can create a more intense orgasm. This can be achieved through hand jobs, oral sex, or using sex toys.

- **Role of the Pelvic Floor Muscles:** Engaging the pelvic floor muscles during anal play can enhance sensations and lead to more powerful orgasms.

- **Breath Control:** Practicing breath control can heighten arousal and increase pleasure during anal and prostate stimulation.

Conclusion

Understanding male anal anatomy is crucial for anyone interested in exploring anal play. By familiarizing yourself with the external and internal structures, particularly the prostate gland, you can enhance your sexual experiences and unlock new levels of pleasure. Remember to prioritize communication, consent, and safety throughout your journey.

In summary, the male anal anatomy offers a wealth of opportunities for exploration and pleasure. Whether you are a novice or an experienced enthusiast, embracing this knowledge can lead to profound sexual satisfaction and a deeper connection with your body and your partner.

External and Internal Structures

Understanding the external and internal structures of male anatomy is crucial for exploring anal pleasure safely and effectively. This section will detail these structures, their functions, and how they can be stimulated to enhance sexual experiences.

External Structures

The external structures of male anatomy relevant to anal play include the anus, perineum, and scrotum.

- **Anus:** The anus is the opening at the end of the digestive tract. It is surrounded by a ring of muscle known as the anal sphincter, which controls the passage of stool and can also provide pleasurable sensations when stimulated. The sensitivity of the anus is due to a high concentration of nerve endings, making it an erogenous zone for many individuals.

- **Perineum:** The perineum is the area between the anus and the scrotum. This region is often referred to as the "taint" and is highly sensitive. Stimulating the perineum can enhance pleasure during anal play and is sometimes referred to as the "male G-spot" due to its proximity to the prostate.

- **Scrotum:** While not directly involved in anal play, the scrotum can be stimulated in tandem with anal activities. The scrotum contains the testicles and is sensitive to touch and pressure, making it an integral part of the male sexual experience.

Internal Structures

The internal structures of the male anatomy that contribute to anal pleasure include the rectum and the prostate gland.

- **Rectum:** The rectum is the final section of the large intestine, leading from the colon to the anus. It is approximately 12 centimeters long and serves as a storage site for fecal matter before excretion. The rectal walls are elastic and can accommodate varying sizes, making it possible to engage in anal play with a range of objects, from fingers to toys. The rectum is also rich in nerve endings, making it sensitive to pressure and stimulation.

- **Prostate Gland:** The prostate is a walnut-sized gland located just below the bladder and in front of the rectum. It plays a key role in male sexual function, producing seminal fluid that nourishes and transports sperm. The prostate can be stimulated through the rectal wall, and many men report that this stimulation can lead to intense orgasms. The prostate is often referred to as the "male G-spot" due to the pleasurable sensations it can provide.

The Role of the Prostate in Pleasure

The prostate can be stimulated through various methods:

1. **Direct Stimulation:** Inserting a finger or a specially designed prostate massager into the rectum can provide direct pressure on the prostate, leading to pleasurable sensations. The ideal position for prostate stimulation is often on the back with knees pulled toward the chest or on all fours.

2. **Indirect Stimulation:** The prostate can also be stimulated indirectly through pressure on the perineum. This method can be particularly pleasurable for individuals who may not be comfortable with direct anal penetration.

3. **Combination Techniques:** Combining anal penetration with stimulation of the penis can enhance the overall experience, as both areas are highly sensitive and can lead to heightened arousal.

Practical Considerations

When engaging in anal play, it is essential to consider the following:

- **Hygiene:** Proper hygiene is crucial for anal play. Cleaning the anal area before engaging in any activities can help prevent infections and enhance comfort. Many individuals choose to use an enema for thorough cleansing, but this is a personal choice and not a necessity for everyone.

- **Lubrication:** The anus does not produce natural lubrication, so using a high-quality lubricant is essential for comfort and pleasure. Silicone-based lubricants are often recommended for anal play due to their long-lasting properties.

- **Communication:** Open and honest communication with partners about comfort levels, boundaries, and desires is vital for a safe and pleasurable experience. Establishing safe words and signals can help ensure that both partners feel secure during play.

Conclusion

Understanding the external and internal structures of male anatomy is foundational for anyone interested in exploring anal pleasure. By recognizing the sensitivity and potential for pleasure in these areas, individuals can enhance their sexual experiences. Always prioritize safety, consent, and communication to ensure a fulfilling exploration of anal play.

The Prostate Gland and Its Role in Pleasure

The prostate gland, often referred to as the male G-spot, is a walnut-sized organ located just below the bladder and in front of the rectum. Its primary function is to produce seminal fluid, which nourishes and transports sperm. However, the prostate is not only significant for reproductive health; it plays a crucial role in male sexual pleasure. Understanding the anatomy and function of the prostate can unlock new dimensions of pleasure for those who explore anal play.

Anatomy of the Prostate

The prostate gland is composed of several zones, each contributing to its function and sensitivity. The main zones are:

- **Peripheral Zone:** This is the largest area of the prostate and is most commonly associated with prostate stimulation. It is located towards the back and is easily accessible through the rectal wall.

- **Central Zone:** This area surrounds the ejaculatory ducts and contributes to seminal fluid production.

- **Transition Zone:** This is the area where benign prostatic hyperplasia (BPH) often occurs, leading to urinary issues in older men.

The prostate is richly supplied with nerve endings, making it highly sensitive to touch and pressure. The proximity of the prostate to the rectal wall means that it can be stimulated through anal penetration, whether by fingers, toys, or during intercourse.

The Role of the Prostate in Pleasure

Stimulation of the prostate can lead to intense sexual arousal and, for some, even orgasm. This phenomenon occurs due to several factors:

- **Nerve Endings:** The prostate is densely packed with nerve endings that can produce pleasurable sensations when stimulated.

- **Fluid Release:** Prostate stimulation can lead to the release of prostatic fluid, which may enhance the experience of ejaculation and increase overall pleasure.

- **Connection to the Pelvic Floor:** The prostate is connected to the pelvic floor muscles, which play a crucial role in sexual arousal and orgasm. Engaging these muscles during stimulation can amplify sensations.

Techniques for Prostate Stimulation

Exploring the prostate can be a thrilling journey, and various techniques can enhance the experience:

Fingers: Using a lubricated finger, gently insert it into the anus and curl it towards the front of the body to locate the prostate. It typically feels like a small, round bump. Experiment with different pressures and rhythms to find what feels best.

Toys: There are many anal toys designed specifically for prostate stimulation. Look for toys that have a curved shape or a bulbous end to target the prostate effectively. Always use plenty of lubrication and start slowly to allow your body to adjust.

Positions: Certain sexual positions can facilitate better access to the prostate. Positions such as doggy style or lying on your back with your legs raised can provide optimal angles for prostate stimulation.

Combining Prostate Stimulation with Other Forms of Pleasure

The experience of prostate stimulation can be enhanced when combined with other forms of sexual pleasure. Here are a few suggestions:

- **Simultaneous Stimulation:** Combine prostate stimulation with other erogenous zones, such as the penis or nipples, to create a more intense experience.

- **Breath Control:** Incorporating breath control techniques can heighten arousal and lead to more powerful orgasms. Experiment with holding your breath or varying your breathing patterns during stimulation.

- **Edging:** Practice edging—bringing yourself close to orgasm and then stopping—can intensify the final release when you do allow yourself to climax.

Common Concerns and Considerations

While exploring prostate stimulation can be pleasurable, there are common concerns that individuals may face:

- **Discomfort:** If you experience pain during prostate stimulation, stop immediately. Discomfort can be a sign of tension or improper technique. Ensure you are relaxed and adequately lubricated.

- **Hygiene:** Maintaining proper hygiene is essential for anal play. Consider using gloves or finger cots and always clean toys before and after use to prevent infections.

- **Communication:** If engaging in anal play with a partner, open communication is vital. Discuss boundaries, desires, and comfort levels to ensure a pleasurable experience for both parties.

Conclusion

The prostate gland is a treasure trove of pleasure waiting to be explored. By understanding its anatomy and how to stimulate it effectively, individuals can enhance their sexual experiences and unlock new levels of enjoyment. Whether through solo exploration or partnered play, embracing the prostate's potential can lead to profound sexual satisfaction. Remember to prioritize consent, communication, and safety as you embark on this exciting journey into anal pleasure.

Techniques for Prostate Stimulation

Prostate stimulation is a powerful avenue for pleasure that can enhance sexual experiences for individuals assigned male at birth. The prostate, often referred to as the "male G-spot," is a walnut-sized gland located approximately two inches inside the rectum, on the anterior wall. This section explores various techniques for prostate stimulation, emphasizing the importance of consent, communication, and safety.

Understanding the Prostate

The prostate gland plays a crucial role in sexual function and pleasure. It produces seminal fluid, which nourishes and transports sperm. Stimulation of the prostate can lead to intense orgasms, often described as more profound than those achieved through penile stimulation alone.

The anatomy of the prostate includes:

- **Location:** The prostate is located about 2-3 inches inside the rectum, towards the front of the body.

- **Size:** Typically the size of a walnut, the prostate can vary in size and sensitivity among individuals.

- **Surrounding Structures:** The prostate is surrounded by nerve endings that can enhance the pleasure experienced during stimulation.

Preparation for Prostate Stimulation

Before engaging in prostate stimulation, it is essential to prepare both mentally and physically. Here are some preparatory steps:

- **Mental Readiness:** Ensure that you are in a comfortable and relaxed state. Consider engaging in deep breathing exercises or mindfulness techniques to enhance relaxation.

- **Physical Preparation:** Clean the anal area thoroughly. Some individuals prefer to use an enema for additional cleanliness, but this is a personal choice.

- **Lubrication:** Use a high-quality water-based or silicone-based lubricant. The anus does not produce natural lubrication, making it crucial to apply ample lubricant to reduce friction and increase comfort.

Basic Techniques for Prostate Stimulation

Once prepared, you can explore various techniques for stimulating the prostate. Here are some effective methods:

UNDERSTANDING THE ANATOMY

1. **Finger Stimulation**

   1. **Positioning:** Start in a comfortable position, such as lying on your back with your legs raised or kneeling with your torso supported.

   2. **Insertion:** Gently insert one or two fingers into the anus, ensuring that you are relaxed and using plenty of lubricant.

   3. **Locate the Prostate:** Curl your fingers towards the front wall of the rectum. You should feel a firm, rounded area—this is the prostate.

   4. **Stimulation:** Use a come-hither motion with your fingers, applying gentle pressure on the prostate. Experiment with different rhythms and pressures to discover what feels best.

2. **Using Prostate Massagers** Prostate massagers are designed specifically for stimulating the prostate. They often have a curved shape and a handle for easy maneuverability.

   1. **Choose the Right Toy:** Select a prostate massager that suits your preferences. Consider size, shape, and vibration features.

   2. **Lubrication:** Apply lubricant generously to both the toy and the anal area.

   3. **Insertion:** Slowly insert the massager, angling it towards the front wall of the rectum to target the prostate.

   4. **Experiment with Settings:** If your massager has vibration settings, experiment with different intensities to find what stimulates you most effectively.

3. **Partner Play** Involving a partner can enhance the experience of prostate stimulation.

   1. **Communication:** Discuss your desires and boundaries with your partner beforehand. Establish safe words to ensure comfort throughout the experience.

   2. **Technique:** Your partner can use their fingers or a prostate massager to stimulate your prostate. Encourage them to explore different angles and pressures.

3. **Combine with Other Stimulation:** Consider combining prostate stimulation with other forms of pleasure, such as oral sex or penile stimulation, for heightened arousal.

Advanced Techniques for Prostate Stimulation

For those seeking to deepen their experience, advanced techniques can be explored.

1. Edging Edging involves bringing yourself close to orgasm and then stopping before climaxing.

1. **Stimulation:** Engage in prostate stimulation while simultaneously stimulating the penis, either through manual techniques or with a toy.

2. **Pause:** When you feel close to orgasm, reduce the intensity or stop stimulation altogether. This can heighten the eventual orgasm when you allow yourself to climax.

2. Combining Anal and Penile Stimulation Simultaneous stimulation of the prostate and penis can create an incredibly intense experience.

1. **Positioning:** Experiment with different positions that allow for both anal and penile stimulation. For example, the doggy style position can facilitate this well.

2. **Rhythm:** Coordinate movements to ensure that both areas receive attention, adjusting the rhythm to maximize pleasure.

Common Challenges and Solutions

While exploring prostate stimulation, some individuals may encounter challenges. Here are common issues and their solutions:

1. Discomfort or Pain

- **Solution:** Ensure adequate lubrication and relaxation. If discomfort persists, stop and reassess your technique. It may also be beneficial to start with smaller toys or fingers.

UNDERSTANDING THE ANATOMY 35

2. Difficulty Locating the Prostate

- **Solution:** Experiment with different angles and positions. Remember that the prostate is located about 2-3 inches inside the rectum and can be more easily accessed when the body is relaxed.

3. Anxiety or Nervousness

- **Solution:** Engage in relaxation techniques before beginning. Open communication with your partner can also alleviate anxiety.

Conclusion

Prostate stimulation can unlock new dimensions of pleasure and intimacy. By understanding the anatomy, preparing adequately, and employing various techniques, individuals can explore their bodies and enhance their sexual experiences. Remember, the key to enjoyable prostate play lies in consent, communication, and a willingness to explore. Embrace your journey into prostate pleasure and enjoy the sensations that await!

Combining Prostate Stimulation with Other Forms of Pleasure

Prostate stimulation is often heralded as a gateway to intense pleasure for those with a prostate. However, combining this experience with other forms of stimulation can elevate the sensations to new heights, creating a symphony of pleasure that resonates throughout the body. In this section, we will explore the theory behind combining prostate stimulation with other forms of pleasure, address potential problems, and provide practical examples to enhance your experience.

Theoretical Framework

The prostate gland, often referred to as the male G-spot, is a walnut-sized organ located about two inches inside the rectum, towards the belly. When stimulated, it can lead to powerful orgasms and heightened sexual arousal. The key to maximizing pleasure lies in understanding the interconnectedness of various erogenous zones and the body's response to multiple forms of stimulation.

$$P = \int_0^T (S_t + E_t)\, dt \tag{7}$$

Where:

- P = Total pleasure experienced
- S_t = Sensation from prostate stimulation at time t
- E_t = Sensation from external stimulation at time t
- T = Duration of the experience

This equation illustrates that the total pleasure P is the integral of sensations from both prostate stimulation S_t and other forms of external stimulation E_t over time T.

Potential Problems

Combining prostate stimulation with other forms of pleasure can lead to a few challenges:

- **Discomfort or Pain:** If one area of stimulation is too intense, it may overshadow the pleasure from prostate stimulation. It's crucial to communicate with your partner and adjust intensity levels accordingly.
- **Distraction:** Focusing on multiple sensations can sometimes lead to confusion or distraction, making it difficult to fully enjoy each type of stimulation. Practicing mindfulness can help maintain focus on the sensations.
- **Safety Concerns:** When using toys or engaging in anal play, safety is paramount. Ensure that all toys are designed for anal use and that proper hygiene practices are followed to avoid infections or injuries.

Practical Examples

To effectively combine prostate stimulation with other forms of pleasure, consider the following techniques:

1. External Stimulation: Engaging in external stimulation, such as clitoral or penile stimulation, while simultaneously stimulating the prostate can create a powerful feedback loop. For example, a partner can use their fingers or a toy to stimulate the prostate while providing external stimulation to the penis or clitoris. This dual approach can enhance arousal and lead to more intense orgasms.

2. **Varying Pressure and Rhythm:** Experiment with varying pressure and rhythm during prostate stimulation. For instance, while one partner focuses on gentle, rhythmic strokes of the prostate, the other can provide varied sensations through oral sex, manual stimulation, or the use of a vibrator. This contrast can create a dynamic interplay of pleasure that keeps the body engaged and responsive.

3. **Incorporating Breath Play:** Breath play can heighten arousal and intensify sensations. Encourage your partner to practice deep, controlled breathing during prostate stimulation. This can help them relax and focus on the sensations. Additionally, incorporating breath-holding techniques can amplify the sensations experienced during orgasm.

4. **Utilizing Toys:** Anal toys designed for prostate stimulation can be paired with other toys for a comprehensive experience. For example, using a vibrating prostate massager while simultaneously stimulating the clitoris with a bullet vibrator can create a multi-layered experience of pleasure. The vibrations can resonate through the body, enhancing the sensations of both forms of stimulation.

5. **Roleplay and Fantasy:** Incorporating roleplay or fantasy scenarios can enhance the overall experience. For example, one partner can take on a dominant role while the other submits, with prostate stimulation serving as a focal point of pleasure. This psychological aspect can deepen the connection and increase arousal, making the physical sensations even more intense.

Conclusion

Combining prostate stimulation with other forms of pleasure is an exciting exploration of the body's capacity for pleasure. By understanding the theoretical underpinnings, addressing potential challenges, and employing practical techniques, individuals can unlock new dimensions of sexual satisfaction. Embrace the journey of discovering what works best for you and your partner, and remember that communication, consent, and creativity are key to a fulfilling experience.

Preparing for Anal Play

Psychological Preparation

The journey into anal play is as much a mental exploration as it is a physical one. Understanding and preparing psychologically can significantly enhance your experience, making it more pleasurable and fulfilling. This section delves into the psychological aspects of anal play, addressing fears, insecurities, and the importance of trust and intimacy.

Understanding Fears and Insecurities

Many individuals harbor fears and insecurities regarding anal play, often stemming from societal stigma, personal experiences, or misconceptions. Common fears include:

- **Pain and Discomfort:** The fear of pain can be a significant barrier. It is crucial to understand that discomfort often arises from tension or lack of preparation. Engaging in relaxation techniques can help alleviate these fears.

- **Judgment:** Concerns about being judged by partners or society can inhibit exploration. Recognizing that pleasure is subjective and personal can empower individuals to embrace their desires.

- **Loss of Control:** The intimate nature of anal play can evoke fears of vulnerability. Establishing boundaries and safe words can provide a sense of control and security.

To address these fears, it is beneficial to engage in self-reflection and open discussions with partners. Journaling thoughts and feelings about anal play can also provide insight and clarity.

Building Trust and Intimacy

Trust is the cornerstone of any intimate relationship, particularly in anal play. Building trust involves:

- **Open Communication:** Discussing desires, boundaries, and fears with your partner fosters a safe environment. Use "I" statements to express your feelings, such as "I feel anxious about trying anal play," which encourages understanding and empathy.

- **Gradual Exploration:** Start with light, non-penetrative activities to build comfort. This could include external stimulation or using fingers to explore the area without pressure to penetrate.

- **Affirmation and Support:** Regularly affirming each other's feelings and experiences can enhance intimacy. Phrases like "I appreciate your openness" or "I'm here for you" reinforce emotional bonds.

Exploring Fantasies and Desires

Understanding your fantasies can illuminate your desires and enhance your anal play experience. Consider the following approaches:

- **Visualization Techniques:** Spend time visualizing scenarios that excite you. This can help clarify what you want to explore and communicate these desires to your partner.

- **Role-Playing:** Engaging in role-play can be a fun way to explore fantasies in a safe environment. Discuss roles and boundaries beforehand to ensure mutual consent and comfort.

- **Reading and Researching:** Explore literature, articles, and forums about anal play to discover what resonates with you. This can also help dispel myths and provide reassurance.

Establishing Boundaries and Limits

Setting boundaries is essential for a fulfilling anal experience. Consider the following steps:

- **Identify Personal Limits:** Reflect on what you are comfortable with and what might be off-limits. This could include specific activities, levels of intensity, or emotional triggers.

- **Create Safe Words:** Establishing safe words provides a clear way to communicate discomfort or the need to pause. Common choices include "red" for stop and "yellow" for slow down.

- **Regular Check-Ins:** During anal play, check in with your partner to ensure both parties are comfortable. Simple questions like "How are you feeling?" can foster ongoing communication.

Conclusion

Psychological preparation is a vital component of successful anal play. By addressing fears, building trust, exploring desires, and establishing boundaries, individuals can create a safe and pleasurable environment for exploration. Remember, the journey into anal pleasure is deeply personal; embrace it with curiosity and an open heart.

Addressing Fears and Insecurities

Engaging in anal play can evoke a range of fears and insecurities, both common and deeply personal. It's essential to acknowledge these feelings, as they can significantly impact your experience and enjoyment. This section aims to explore the roots of these fears, offer strategies for overcoming them, and empower you to embrace your desires fully.

Understanding the Roots of Fear

Fears surrounding anal play often stem from societal stigma, personal beliefs, and past experiences. Common fears include:

- **Fear of Pain:** Many individuals worry that anal play will be painful or uncomfortable. This fear can be exacerbated by misconceptions about anal anatomy and the lack of proper preparation.

- **Fear of Judgment:** Concerns about how others perceive anal play can create significant anxiety. Many people internalize societal taboos, leading to feelings of shame or guilt.

- **Fear of Loss of Control:** The intimate nature of anal play can provoke fears about vulnerability and losing control during the experience. This fear can be particularly pronounced in those who have experienced trauma or abuse.

- **Fear of Physical Reactions:** Some individuals worry about involuntary bodily reactions, such as incontinence or discomfort, which can deter them from exploring anal play.

Strategies for Overcoming Fears

Addressing these fears involves a combination of education, communication, and self-reflection. Here are some strategies to help you navigate your insecurities:

1. Education and Awareness Knowledge is power. Understanding the anatomy involved in anal play, as well as the techniques for safe and pleasurable experiences, can alleviate fears. For instance, learning about the importance of relaxation, lubrication, and gradual exploration can help mitigate concerns about pain.

2. Open Communication Discussing your fears with your partner(s) is crucial. Open dialogues can foster trust and understanding, allowing you to express your concerns and desires without judgment. For example, you might say, "I'm feeling a bit anxious about trying anal play. Can we take it slow and check in with each other regularly?"

3. Gradual Exposure Start with small steps to build your comfort level. This might include exploring external anal stimulation before progressing to penetration. Gradual exposure can help desensitize fears and create a more positive association with anal play.

4. Mindfulness and Relaxation Techniques Incorporating mindfulness practices, such as deep breathing or meditation, can help you manage anxiety. Before engaging in anal play, take a few moments to center yourself and focus on your body's sensations. This can create a more relaxed state, making it easier to explore.

5. Positive Affirmations Challenge negative thoughts with positive affirmations. Remind yourself of your right to pleasure and the importance of consent. Phrases like "I am in control of my body" or "I deserve to explore my desires" can be empowering.

Examples of Overcoming Fears

Consider the following scenarios that illustrate how individuals can address their fears:

Example 1: Pain Anxiety Sarah has always been curious about anal play but is terrified of the pain she has heard about. After researching and learning about the importance of relaxation and lubrication, she decides to communicate her fears to her partner. Together, they agree to start with external stimulation and use plenty of lubricant, allowing Sarah to control the pace. By taking it slow, she discovers that with proper preparation, anal play can be pleasurable rather than painful.

Example 2: Fear of Judgment Michael has always felt embarrassed about his interest in anal play due to societal stigma. After joining a supportive online community, he learns that many others share similar interests and fears. Encouraged by this newfound perspective, he opens up to his partner about his desires. To his relief, she is supportive and willing to explore together, alleviating his fear of judgment.

Example 3: Loss of Control Jessica has experienced trauma in the past, leading to a fear of losing control during anal play. To address this, she engages in open discussions with her partner about her boundaries and safe words. They establish a clear plan for their exploration, allowing Jessica to feel secure. By prioritizing communication and consent, she gradually builds trust and confidence in her ability to navigate her fears.

Conclusion

Addressing fears and insecurities is a vital part of the journey toward embracing anal play. By understanding the roots of your fears, employing effective strategies, and communicating openly with your partner(s), you can create a safe and pleasurable experience. Remember, your desires are valid, and with patience and practice, you can unlock the pleasures that anal play has to offer.

Building Trust and Intimacy

Building trust and intimacy is a fundamental aspect of any sexual relationship, especially when exploring anal play. The unique nature of anal play can evoke a range of emotions, from excitement to apprehension. Therefore, creating a safe and trusting environment is essential for both partners to fully enjoy the experience. This section delves into the importance of trust and intimacy, the challenges that may arise, and practical strategies to foster these essential elements.

The Importance of Trust

Trust serves as the foundation for any intimate relationship. It allows partners to feel secure, respected, and valued. In the context of anal play, trust becomes even more critical due to the physical and emotional vulnerabilities involved. When partners trust each other, they can communicate openly about their desires, fears, and boundaries without fear of judgment or rejection.

Challenges to Trust

Despite its importance, building trust can be challenging. Factors that may hinder trust-building include:

- **Past Experiences:** Previous negative experiences with anal play or intimacy can create barriers to trust. If one partner has faced pain or trauma, it may lead to hesitance in exploring anal play again.

- **Societal Stigma:** The stigma surrounding anal play can lead to feelings of shame or embarrassment, making it difficult for partners to discuss their desires openly.

- **Fear of Judgment:** Partners may worry about being judged for their interests or preferences, which can stifle honest communication.

- **Insecurity:** Personal insecurities related to body image or sexual performance can inhibit a partner's willingness to engage in anal play.

Strategies for Building Trust

To overcome these challenges and foster trust, consider the following strategies:

1. Open Communication Establishing a habit of open communication is vital. Discuss your interests, boundaries, and concerns regarding anal play. Use "I" statements to express your feelings and desires, such as "I feel excited about trying anal play, but I'm also a bit nervous." This approach minimizes defensiveness and encourages understanding.

2. Establish Safe Words Creating safe words is a powerful way to enhance trust. A safe word is a pre-agreed term that either partner can use to pause or stop the activity. This ensures that both partners feel secure in their ability to communicate discomfort or the need for a break. Common safe words include "red" for stop and "yellow" for slow down.

3. Gradual Exploration Take your time when exploring anal play. Start with lighter forms of stimulation, such as external anal massage or using fingers, before moving on to more intense activities. This gradual approach allows both partners to build confidence and comfort with each step.

4. Mutual Consent and Agreement   Ensure that both partners enthusiastically consent to engage in anal play. Consent should be ongoing and can be revoked at any time. Discuss what each partner is comfortable with and establish clear boundaries. This process reinforces respect for each other's limits and desires.

5. Create a Safe Environment   A safe physical and emotional environment is crucial for building intimacy. Choose a comfortable space where both partners feel relaxed and free from interruptions. Dim lighting, soft music, and comfortable bedding can enhance the atmosphere and promote intimacy.

6. Engage in Aftercare   Aftercare is an essential component of any intimate experience, particularly after anal play. It involves caring for each other emotionally and physically post-activity. This can include cuddling, discussing the experience, or simply lying together in silence. Aftercare helps reinforce the bond between partners and demonstrates commitment to each other's well-being.

Examples of Building Trust and Intimacy

To illustrate these strategies, consider the following scenarios:

Scenario 1: Open Communication   Jessica and Alex are considering anal play for the first time. They sit down together and discuss their feelings about it. Jessica expresses her excitement but also shares her fear of pain. Alex listens attentively, reassures her, and shares his own feelings of nervousness. Together, they agree to start slowly and check in with each other throughout the experience.

Scenario 2: Establishing Safe Words   During their conversation, Jessica and Alex agree on safe words. They choose "red" to indicate an immediate stop and "yellow" to signal that they need to slow down. This agreement fosters a sense of security, knowing that they can communicate their limits at any time.

Scenario 3: Gradual Exploration   On the day of their planned anal play, Jessica and Alex begin with a sensual massage. They explore each other's bodies, gradually moving towards anal stimulation. They start with light external massage around the anal area, allowing Jessica to adjust to the sensations before any penetration occurs.

Scenario 4: Aftercare After their intimate experience, Jessica and Alex engage in aftercare. They cuddle under a blanket, share their thoughts about what they enjoyed, and discuss any discomfort that may have arisen. This debriefing strengthens their emotional connection and reassures them both that their feelings are valid.

Conclusion

Building trust and intimacy is a continuous process that requires effort and commitment from both partners. By prioritizing open communication, establishing safe words, and creating a supportive environment, couples can enhance their anal play experiences. Remember, trust is not built overnight; it evolves through shared experiences, understanding, and mutual respect. Embrace the journey of building trust and intimacy as a vital part of your exploration into anal pleasure, and celebrate the deepening connection it fosters between you and your partner.

Exploring Fantasies and Desires

Exploring fantasies and desires is a crucial aspect of sexual expression, especially when it comes to anal play. Understanding what excites you and your partner can lead to deeper intimacy and enhanced pleasure. This section will guide you through the process of identifying, communicating, and embracing your fantasies and desires.

The Nature of Fantasies

Fantasies are imaginative scenarios that often reflect our deepest desires and curiosities. They can range from the mundane to the extraordinary, encompassing a wide array of themes, including power dynamics, roleplay, and the exploration of taboo subjects. The psychological basis of fantasies can be understood through several theories:

- **Psychodynamic Theory:** Sigmund Freud posited that fantasies are manifestations of repressed desires. In this view, engaging with fantasies allows individuals to explore aspects of their psyche that may be socially unacceptable.

- **Cognitive Theory:** This theory suggests that fantasies serve as a form of cognitive rehearsal, allowing individuals to mentally explore scenarios that they may not be ready to pursue in reality.

- **Humanistic Theory:** This perspective emphasizes the importance of personal growth and self-actualization. Fantasies can be seen as pathways to understanding oneself and fulfilling one's potential for pleasure and intimacy.

Identifying Your Fantasies

To explore your fantasies, start by engaging in self-reflection. Consider the following questions:

1. What scenarios excite you?

2. Are there particular themes or dynamics that appeal to you, such as dominance and submission, or role reversals?

3. How do you feel about the idea of anal play? Does it evoke curiosity, excitement, fear, or a combination of emotions?

Writing down your thoughts can help clarify your desires. You might also consider keeping a journal dedicated to your sexual fantasies. This practice not only aids in self-discovery but can also serve as a tool for communication with your partner.

Communicating Fantasies with Your Partner

Once you've identified your fantasies, the next step is to communicate them to your partner. Open and honest dialogue is vital for establishing trust and ensuring that both partners feel safe and respected. Here are some tips for effective communication:

- **Choose the Right Time:** Initiate the conversation in a relaxed setting where both partners feel comfortable discussing their desires without distractions.

- **Use "I" Statements:** Frame your desires from your perspective. For example, say "I fantasize about..." rather than "You should...". This approach fosters a non-confrontational atmosphere.

- **Be Open to Feedback:** Encourage your partner to share their fantasies as well. This mutual exchange can deepen intimacy and create a safe space for exploration.

PREPARING FOR ANAL PLAY

Embracing Your Desires

Embracing your fantasies means accepting them without shame or judgment. It is essential to recognize that desires are a natural part of human sexuality. Here are some strategies for embracing your desires:

- **Practice Self-Acceptance:** Acknowledge that your fantasies are valid and a part of who you are. Engage in positive self-talk and remind yourself that exploring your desires can lead to personal growth.

- **Explore Gradually:** If your fantasies involve elements that seem daunting, consider exploring them gradually. Start with less intense scenarios and build up to more adventurous experiences as you and your partner become more comfortable.

- **Incorporate Safe Words:** Establish safe words to ensure that both partners can communicate their comfort levels during exploration. This practice reinforces trust and makes it easier to navigate boundaries.

Examples of Fantasies Related to Anal Play

To inspire your exploration, here are some common fantasies related to anal play:

- **Power Dynamics:** Many individuals fantasize about the exchange of power during anal play, where one partner takes on a dominant role while the other submits. This can enhance the experience by adding an element of excitement and psychological stimulation.

- **Roleplay Scenarios:** Engaging in roleplay can heighten arousal. Consider scenarios like a doctor-patient dynamic or a teacher-student relationship, where anal play becomes part of the fantasy narrative.

- **Public or Semi-Public Settings:** Some may fantasize about being intimate in a public or semi-public space, which can add an exhilarating sense of risk and excitement to anal play.

Addressing Fears and Concerns

While exploring fantasies can be thrilling, it is not uncommon to encounter fears or concerns. Addressing these feelings is crucial for a fulfilling experience:

- **Fear of Judgment:** It's natural to worry about how your fantasies may be perceived. Remember that everyone has unique desires, and open communication with your partner can help alleviate these fears.

- **Concerns about Safety:** If your fantasies involve elements that could pose physical or emotional risks, prioritize safety. Discuss boundaries, establish safe words, and ensure that both partners are informed about safety precautions.

- **Emotional Vulnerability:** Engaging in fantasies can evoke strong emotions. Be prepared for the possibility of unexpected feelings arising during exploration and establish a debriefing process to discuss experiences afterward.

Conclusion

Exploring fantasies and desires is an empowering journey that can enrich your sexual experiences and deepen your connection with your partner. By understanding the nature of your fantasies, communicating openly, and embracing your desires, you can unlock a world of pleasure and intimacy. Remember, the key to a fulfilling exploration lies in mutual respect, consent, and a willingness to navigate the exciting terrain of your sexual landscape together.

Establishing Boundaries and Limits

Establishing boundaries and limits is a fundamental aspect of engaging in anal play, ensuring that all participants feel safe, respected, and empowered. This section will delve into the importance of boundaries, the various types of limits, and practical strategies to communicate and enforce them effectively.

Understanding Boundaries

Boundaries are the personal guidelines that define what is acceptable and what is not in any sexual encounter. They serve to protect individual comfort levels and emotional well-being, allowing for a consensual and pleasurable experience. In anal play, boundaries can encompass physical, emotional, and psychological aspects.

Types of Boundaries

- **Physical Boundaries:** These pertain to the types of physical contact that are acceptable. For instance, some individuals may be comfortable with external anal stimulation but not with penetration.

- **Emotional Boundaries:** These relate to how individuals feel during the experience. It's essential to discuss any emotional triggers or past experiences that may affect the current encounter.

- **Psychological Boundaries:** These involve mental comfort and safety, particularly regarding fantasies, roleplay, and power dynamics. Consent should be enthusiastic and ongoing.

The Importance of Communication

Effective communication is vital in establishing boundaries. It is essential to have open discussions before engaging in anal play, where all parties can express their desires, fears, and limits without fear of judgment. This dialogue can involve the following steps:

1. **Initiate the Conversation:** Approach the topic of anal play with your partner(s) in a relaxed setting. Use open-ended questions to encourage dialogue, such as, "What are your thoughts on trying anal play?"

2. **Share Personal Limits:** Be honest about your boundaries. For example, you might say, "I'm interested in trying anal play, but I'm not comfortable with fisting."

3. **Listen Actively:** Pay attention to your partner's responses and validate their feelings. If they express discomfort, respect their boundaries without pressure.

4. **Negotiate:** Find common ground. If one partner is unsure about a specific act, discuss alternatives that respect both parties' limits.

Establishing Safe Words and Signals

A critical component of boundary-setting is the establishment of safe words and signals. These are predetermined words or gestures that can be used to pause or stop the activity if someone feels uncomfortable or overwhelmed.

- **Safe Words:** Choose simple, easy-to-remember words that are unlikely to come up in normal conversation. Common examples include "red" for stop, "yellow" for slow down, and "green" for continue.

- **Non-Verbal Signals:** In situations where verbal communication may be difficult, establish non-verbal signals, such as a hand squeeze or a specific gesture.

Respecting Personal Boundaries

Respecting boundaries is not just about acknowledging them; it is about actively ensuring they are upheld throughout the experience. This involves:

- **Checking In:** Regularly check in with your partner(s) during anal play. Simple questions like, "How are you feeling?" or "Is this still okay?" can help maintain a safe environment.

- **Observing Body Language:** Pay attention to non-verbal cues. If your partner appears tense or withdrawn, pause and discuss their comfort level.

- **Being Prepared to Stop:** If a boundary is crossed, be ready to halt the activity immediately. This demonstrates respect for your partner's limits and reinforces trust.

Debriefing and Aftercare

Aftercare is a crucial part of the anal play experience, especially when exploring intense sensations or pushing boundaries. Aftercare involves checking in with each other post-activity to discuss feelings, experiences, and any discomfort that may have arisen.

- **Discuss the Experience:** Talk about what was enjoyable and what may have been uncomfortable. This feedback loop can enhance future encounters.

- **Provide Comfort:** Engage in comforting activities, such as cuddling or gentle touch, to reinforce emotional safety and connection.

- **Reflect on Boundaries:** Use this time to reassess boundaries. Are there new limits that need to be established? Did the experience change any perspectives?

PREPARING FOR ANAL PLAY

Conclusion

Establishing boundaries and limits is an empowering process that enhances the experience of anal play. By fostering open communication, respecting personal limits, and engaging in aftercare, individuals can create a safe and pleasurable environment that celebrates their desires. Remember, the journey of exploration is ongoing, and boundaries may evolve as comfort and trust grow. Embrace the dialogue, and let it guide you toward deeper intimacy and pleasure.

Physical Preparation

Physical preparation is a crucial aspect of anal play, as it ensures that both partners feel comfortable and ready for the experience. This section will cover various elements of physical preparation, including hygiene practices, lubrication techniques, pelvic floor muscle strengthening, and stretching and relaxation exercises.

Hygiene Practices

Maintaining proper hygiene is essential for a safe and enjoyable anal experience. Here are some key practices to consider:

- **Cleaning the Anal Area:** Use mild soap and water to clean the anal region thoroughly. Some individuals may prefer to use a bulb syringe or an enema for internal cleaning, but this is a personal choice and should be approached with caution. If you choose to use an enema, ensure that you follow the instructions carefully to avoid any discomfort or injury.

- **Nail Care:** If using fingers for anal play, it is vital to keep nails trimmed and smooth to prevent any scratches or tears. Consider using a nail file to smooth out any sharp edges.

- **Personal Grooming:** While not necessary for everyone, some individuals prefer to groom the anal area for aesthetic or comfort reasons. This can include shaving or trimming pubic hair, but it is essential to do so carefully to avoid irritation or ingrown hairs.

Lubrication Techniques

Lubrication is key to ensuring a pleasurable anal experience. The anus does not self-lubricate, making the use of a high-quality lubricant essential. Here are some considerations:

- **Types of Lubricants:** There are several types of lubricants available, including water-based, silicone-based, and oil-based options. Each has its pros and cons:
  - *Water-based lubricants* are easy to clean, safe to use with condoms and toys, but may require reapplication.
  - *Silicone-based lubricants* last longer and provide a silky feel but should not be used with silicone toys.
  - *Oil-based lubricants* can provide excellent glide but are not safe with latex condoms and can be more challenging to clean.
- **Applying Lubricant:** Generously apply lubricant to both the anus and any inserting fingers or toys. Ensure that there is sufficient lubrication throughout the entire experience to prevent discomfort.

Strengthening the Pelvic Floor Muscles

Strong pelvic floor muscles can enhance anal play by promoting relaxation and control. Here are some exercises to consider:

- **Kegel Exercises:** These exercises involve contracting and relaxing the pelvic floor muscles. To perform a Kegel, identify the muscles used to stop urination. Contract these muscles for five seconds, then relax for five seconds. Repeat this process 10-15 times, three times a day. Gradually increase the duration of the contractions as your strength improves.
- **Bridge Pose:** This yoga pose not only strengthens the pelvic floor but also engages the glutes and lower back. To perform a bridge, lie on your back with your knees bent and feet flat on the floor. Lift your hips toward the ceiling while squeezing your glutes and pelvic floor muscles. Hold for a few seconds, then lower back down. Repeat 10-15 times.

Stretching and Relaxation Exercises

Incorporating stretching and relaxation exercises can help alleviate tension and prepare the body for anal play. Here are some techniques:

- **Deep Breathing:** Deep, controlled breathing can promote relaxation and reduce anxiety. Inhale deeply through the nose, allowing the abdomen to expand, and then exhale slowly through the mouth. Repeat this for several minutes to create a sense of calm.

- **Gentle Stretching:** Incorporate gentle stretches to relax the muscles around the anus. For instance, while lying on your back, bring your knees to your chest and gently rock side to side. This can help release tension in the lower back and pelvic area.
- **Butterfly Stretch:** Sit with the soles of your feet together and gently press your knees toward the floor. This stretch opens up the hips and promotes relaxation in the pelvic region.

Conclusion

Physical preparation is an integral part of anal play that can significantly enhance the experience. By prioritizing hygiene, using appropriate lubrication, strengthening the pelvic floor muscles, and incorporating stretching and relaxation techniques, individuals can create a safe and pleasurable environment for exploration. Remember, the key to a fulfilling anal experience lies in preparation, communication, and mutual consent. Embrace the journey and enjoy the pleasures that await!

Hygiene Practices

When it comes to anal play, hygiene is paramount. Proper hygiene not only enhances the experience but also minimizes health risks. This section will explore essential hygiene practices for anal play, ensuring that both partners feel safe, comfortable, and ready to explore their desires.

Understanding the Importance of Hygiene

The anus is a sensitive area that can harbor bacteria. Proper cleaning before engaging in anal play can prevent infections and ensure a pleasurable experience. The rectum contains a variety of bacteria, some of which can lead to infections if introduced into the vaginal canal or bloodstream. Therefore, understanding and implementing effective hygiene practices is crucial.

Pre-Play Hygiene

- **Bowel Movement:** Before engaging in anal play, it is advisable to have a bowel movement. This not only reduces the risk of fecal matter interfering with the experience but also helps you feel more relaxed and confident.

- **Washing:** A thorough wash of the anal area with warm water and mild soap is recommended. It is essential to rinse well to avoid any soap residue, which can cause irritation.

- **Enemas:** Some individuals choose to use enemas for additional cleansing. If you opt for an enema, it is crucial to use it correctly. A bulb syringe or a bag enema can be used, but be sure to follow the instructions carefully. Using distilled or filtered water is recommended to avoid introducing harmful bacteria. Note that overuse of enemas can irritate the rectal lining, so they should be used sparingly.

During Play Hygiene

Maintaining hygiene during anal play is equally important. Here are some practices to consider:

- **Gloves:** Wearing latex or nitrile gloves can help maintain cleanliness and reduce the risk of transferring bacteria. This is particularly important if you are using fingers or toys.

- **Lubrication:** Use a high-quality lubricant that is safe for anal play. Avoid oil-based lubricants if you are using condoms, as they can degrade the material. Water-based or silicone-based lubricants are recommended for anal play.

- **Toys:** If using anal toys, ensure they are cleaned properly before and after use. Use warm water and soap or a dedicated toy cleaner. Always check that the toy is in good condition, with no cracks or damage that could harbor bacteria.

Post-Play Hygiene

After engaging in anal play, it is essential to follow up with proper hygiene practices:

- **Washing:** Both partners should wash their hands and any body parts that came into contact with the anal area. This helps to prevent the spread of bacteria and ensures cleanliness.

- **Cleaning Toys:** Clean all toys used during anal play immediately after use. This ensures that any bacteria are eliminated and prevents contamination for future sessions.

- **Monitoring for Discomfort:** After anal play, be attentive to any signs of discomfort or irritation. If you experience any unusual symptoms, such as persistent pain, bleeding, or unusual discharge, consult a healthcare provider.

Common Hygiene Challenges

While maintaining hygiene during anal play is essential, some challenges may arise:

- **Embarrassment:** Some individuals may feel embarrassed discussing hygiene with their partner. Open communication about hygiene practices can help alleviate discomfort and foster a more trusting environment.
- **Time Constraints:** In the heat of the moment, hygiene practices may be overlooked. Setting aside dedicated time for preparation can help ensure that both partners feel comfortable and ready for play.
- **Sensitivity and Irritation:** Some individuals may have sensitive skin that reacts to soaps or lubricants. Testing products on a small area of skin before use can help identify any potential irritants.

Conclusion

In conclusion, hygiene practices are a crucial component of anal play. By prioritizing cleanliness before, during, and after play, you can enhance the experience and minimize health risks. Open communication with your partner about hygiene preferences and practices can also foster trust and intimacy, allowing you to fully embrace your anal journey.

By understanding and implementing these hygiene practices, you can create a safe and pleasurable environment for exploring anal play. Remember, a clean slate leads to a more enjoyable experience, so take the time to ensure that both you and your partner are ready to dive into the depths of pleasure without hesitation.

Lubrication Techniques

When it comes to anal play, lubrication is not merely a suggestion; it is a necessity. The anus does not produce its own lubrication, making the use of additional products essential for comfort, pleasure, and safety. This section will explore various lubrication techniques, the types of lubricants available, their properties, and how to effectively apply them to enhance your anal experience.

Understanding Lubricants

Lubricants can be classified into three main categories: water-based, silicone-based, and oil-based. Each type has its unique properties and uses.

- **Water-Based Lubricants:** These are versatile and easy to clean up. They are safe to use with condoms and most sex toys. However, they can dry out quickly, requiring reapplication. An example is *Astroglide*, which provides a smooth glide and is easily washable.

- **Silicone-Based Lubricants:** These offer a longer-lasting glide compared to water-based options and are also safe for use with condoms. They can be used in water, making them ideal for shower or bath play. However, they should not be used with silicone toys, as they can degrade the material. A popular choice is *Pjur*, known for its silky texture and longevity.

- **Oil-Based Lubricants:** These provide a luxurious feel and are great for massages and prolonged play. However, they should not be used with latex condoms as they can cause breakage. Examples include coconut oil and *Bert's Bees*, which are natural and provide a soothing effect on the skin.

Choosing the Right Lubricant

Selecting the right lubricant is crucial for a pleasurable anal experience. Consider the following factors:

1. **Sensitivity:** If you or your partner have sensitive skin, opt for hypoallergenic water-based lubricants that are free from fragrances and irritants.

2. **Duration of Play:** For longer sessions, silicone-based lubricants are preferable due to their longevity. For shorter encounters, water-based lubricants may suffice.

3. **Type of Play:** If incorporating toys, ensure the lubricant is compatible with the material of the toy. For example, avoid silicone-based lubricants with silicone toys.

Application Techniques

Effective application of lubricant can significantly enhance the experience. Here are some techniques to consider:

- **Generous Application:** Start with a generous amount of lubricant on your fingers or the toy. This ensures that the initial contact is smooth and comfortable.

- **Layering:** For additional comfort, apply lubricant both externally and internally. Start by massaging the anal area with lubricant to relax the sphincter muscles before attempting penetration.

- **Reapplication:** Be prepared to reapply lubricant as needed. If you notice any friction or discomfort, stop and add more lubricant. Listening to your body is key.

- **Temperature Play:** Experiment with warming the lubricant in your hands before application. Some individuals enjoy the sensation of warm lubricant, which can enhance relaxation and arousal.

Common Problems and Solutions

Even with the best intentions, issues can arise during anal play. Here are some common problems and solutions related to lubrication:

- **Dryness:** If you experience dryness during play, pause and apply more lubricant. Consider switching to a silicone-based lubricant for longer-lasting moisture.

- **Irritation:** If irritation occurs, discontinue use of the lubricant immediately. Opt for a hypoallergenic formula for future sessions.

- **Incompatibility:** If using condoms, ensure the lubricant is compatible. Oil-based lubricants can cause latex condoms to break, leading to potential risks.

Conclusion

In conclusion, lubrication is a fundamental aspect of anal play that should not be overlooked. By understanding the different types of lubricants, selecting the appropriate one, and applying it effectively, you can enhance your experience and ensure comfort and safety. Remember, the key to pleasurable anal play is communication with your partner, so don't hesitate to discuss your lubrication preferences and needs. Embrace the power of lubrication and unlock the gateway to extreme pleasure.

$$\text{Pleasure} = \text{Communication} + \text{Preparation} + \text{Lubrication} \qquad (8)$$

Strengthening the Pelvic Floor Muscles

The pelvic floor is a crucial area of the body that supports the pelvic organs, including the bladder, intestines, and, in women, the uterus. Strengthening these muscles can enhance sexual pleasure, improve control during anal play, and contribute to overall sexual health.

Anatomy of the Pelvic Floor

The pelvic floor consists of a group of muscles and connective tissues that form a supportive hammock across the bottom of the pelvis. These muscles include:

- **Pubococcygeus (PC) Muscle:** This muscle supports the pelvic organs and plays a significant role in sexual function.
- **Iliococcygeus Muscle:** This muscle helps in maintaining pelvic stability.
- **Coccygeus Muscle:** It supports the coccyx and contributes to the overall strength of the pelvic floor.

Importance of Strengthening the Pelvic Floor

Strengthening the pelvic floor muscles has several benefits:

- **Increased Sexual Pleasure:** Strong pelvic floor muscles can enhance orgasm intensity and control during anal play.
- **Improved Bladder and Bowel Control:** A strong pelvic floor helps prevent urinary incontinence and supports bowel function.
- **Enhanced Support for Pelvic Organs:** Strong muscles help maintain the proper position of pelvic organs, reducing the risk of prolapse.

Common Problems Associated with Weak Pelvic Floor Muscles

Weak pelvic floor muscles can lead to various issues, such as:

- **Urinary Incontinence:** Involuntary leakage of urine during activities like coughing, sneezing, or exercise.

- **Pelvic Organ Prolapse:** A condition where pelvic organs descend into the vaginal canal due to insufficient support.

- **Decreased Sexual Pleasure:** Weak muscles can result in diminished sensation and control during sexual activities.

Exercises for Strengthening the Pelvic Floor

Several exercises can effectively strengthen the pelvic floor muscles. The most well-known is the Kegel exercise, which can be performed by both men and women.

Kegel Exercises To perform Kegel exercises:

1. Identify the pelvic floor muscles by attempting to stop urination mid-flow. The muscles you use are your pelvic floor muscles.

2. Once identified, empty your bladder and find a comfortable position (lying down, sitting, or standing).

3. Tighten your pelvic floor muscles and hold the contraction for **3 to 5 seconds**.

4. Relax the muscles for the same amount of time.

5. Repeat this process **10 to 15 times** in one session.

6. Aim for **three sessions** per day.

Advanced Techniques As strength improves, you can advance your Kegel exercises by incorporating variations:

- **Quick Flicks:** Rapidly contract and relax the pelvic floor muscles for **10 to 15 repetitions**. This helps improve muscle responsiveness.

- **Weighted Kegels:** Use vaginal weights designed for pelvic floor training to add resistance and increase the challenge of the exercises.

Incorporating Pelvic Floor Exercises into Your Routine

To maximize the benefits of pelvic floor exercises, consider the following tips:

- **Consistency is Key:** Make pelvic floor exercises a regular part of your daily routine.

- **Mindfulness:** Focus on the contraction and relaxation of the pelvic floor muscles to enhance awareness and effectiveness.

- **Breathing Techniques:** Incorporate deep breathing while performing exercises to promote relaxation and enhance muscle engagement.

Monitoring Progress and Results

It is essential to monitor your progress as you strengthen your pelvic floor muscles. Signs of improvement may include:

- Increased control during anal play and sexual activities.

- Enhanced sensation and intensity of orgasms.

- Improved bladder control and reduced instances of leakage.

Consider keeping a journal to track your exercises, feelings, and any changes in your sexual experiences. This reflection can help reinforce your commitment and provide insight into your progress.

Conclusion

Strengthening the pelvic floor muscles is a vital component of enhancing sexual pleasure and improving overall sexual health. By incorporating targeted exercises, such as Kegel exercises, into your routine, you can unlock new dimensions of pleasure in your anal play journey. Remember, consistency and mindfulness are crucial for achieving the best results. Embrace the journey of strengthening your pelvic floor and discover the empowering benefits it brings to your sexual experiences.

Stretching and Relaxation Exercises

Stretching and relaxation exercises are essential components of preparing for anal play. They help to alleviate tension, increase flexibility, and enhance overall comfort, making the experience more pleasurable. This section will explore various techniques, their theoretical foundations, and practical applications.

The Importance of Stretching

Stretching serves multiple purposes in the context of anal play:

- **Increased Flexibility:** Regular stretching can improve the flexibility of the anal sphincter muscles, making it easier to accommodate penetration.

- **Reduced Tension:** Stretching helps to release physical tension in the body, particularly in the pelvic region, which can be a common area of stress and tightness.

- **Enhanced Circulation:** Improved blood flow to the area can heighten sensitivity and arousal, enhancing the overall experience.

Basic Stretching Techniques

Here are some effective stretching exercises to incorporate into your preparation routine:

1. The Butterfly Stretch

1. Sit on the floor with your back straight.
2. Bring the soles of your feet together, allowing your knees to drop outward.
3. Gently press your knees toward the floor using your elbows for a deeper stretch.
4. Hold this position for 30 seconds, breathing deeply.

2. The Seated Forward Bend

1. Sit with your legs extended in front of you.
2. Inhale deeply, raising your arms overhead.

3. Exhale as you bend forward at the hips, reaching for your toes.

4. Hold for 30 seconds, focusing on relaxing your lower back and hips.

3. The Cat-Cow Stretch

1. Start on all fours with your wrists under your shoulders and knees under your hips.

2. Inhale as you arch your back (Cat), lifting your head and tailbone.

3. Exhale as you round your back (Cow), tucking your chin to your chest.

4. Repeat for 5 cycles, synchronizing your breath with your movements.

Relaxation Techniques

In addition to stretching, relaxation exercises are crucial for easing anxiety and preparing mentally for anal play.

1. Deep Breathing

- Find a comfortable position, either sitting or lying down.
- Inhale deeply through your nose, allowing your abdomen to expand.
- Hold the breath for a moment, then exhale slowly through your mouth.
- Repeat for 5-10 minutes, focusing on the rhythm of your breath.

2. Progressive Muscle Relaxation

1. Lie down in a quiet space, closing your eyes.

2. Starting from your toes, tense each muscle group for 5 seconds, then release.

3. Move upward through your body, focusing on areas of tension, including the pelvic region.

4. Take a moment to notice the difference between tension and relaxation.

Addressing Common Problems

While stretching and relaxation can enhance anal play, some individuals may encounter challenges:

- **Discomfort or Pain:** If you experience pain during stretching, ease back and only stretch to a comfortable point. Pain is a signal that you may be pushing too hard.
- **Difficulty Relaxing:** Anxiety can hinder relaxation. Consider incorporating calming music or guided meditation to help ease your mind.
- **Inconsistent Practice:** Regular practice is key to seeing improvements in flexibility and relaxation. Aim to incorporate these exercises into your routine at least 2-3 times a week.

Example Routine

To help you integrate stretching and relaxation into your preparation, here's a simple routine you can follow:

1. **Warm-Up:** 5 minutes of light cardio (e.g., walking or gentle dancing).
2. **Stretching:** Perform each of the stretching exercises listed above, holding each for 30 seconds.
3. **Deep Breathing:** 5-10 minutes of deep breathing exercises.
4. **Progressive Muscle Relaxation:** 5-10 minutes focusing on relaxing each muscle group.

Incorporating these stretching and relaxation exercises into your anal play preparation can significantly enhance your experience. By fostering a state of physical and mental readiness, you can embrace the pleasures that await you with confidence and joy.

Conclusion

Stretching and relaxation are vital components of a fulfilling anal play experience. By prioritizing these practices, you can overcome physical barriers, reduce anxiety, and create a space for exploration and pleasure. Remember, the journey to unlocking extreme pleasure begins with a relaxed body and an open mind.

Basic Anal Techniques

Finger Techniques

Finger techniques are foundational to exploring anal pleasure, offering a pathway to understanding both personal desires and the anatomy involved. This section delves into the various methods of finger stimulation, safety considerations, and how to enhance pleasure for both partners.

The Basics of Finger Techniques

Engaging in anal play with fingers requires a delicate balance of comfort, trust, and communication. The fingers can be used for exploration, stimulation, and preparation, making them versatile tools for both solo and partner play.

Anatomical Considerations

Before diving into techniques, it's crucial to understand the anatomy involved. The anal area is rich in nerve endings, making it highly sensitive. The external anal sphincter, located around the anal opening, can be stimulated directly. Internally, the rectum and surrounding structures, including the prostate in males and the G-spot in females, can be targeted through careful finger placement.

Preparation and Hygiene

Prior to engaging in anal play, ensure that both partners are comfortable and informed. This includes:

- **Hygiene:** Wash hands thoroughly and trim nails to avoid injury. Consider wearing gloves for added safety and ease of cleanup.

- **Lubrication:** Use a generous amount of lubricant, as the anal area does not produce natural lubrication. Water-based or silicone-based lubes are recommended.

- **Communication:** Discuss boundaries, desires, and safe words before starting. Ensure that both partners feel safe and respected.

BASIC ANAL TECHNIQUES   67

Techniques for Anal Finger Play

1. The Teasing Touch   Start with gentle external stimulation. Use the fingertips to circle around the anal opening, applying varying pressure. This technique helps relax the sphincter and build anticipation.

2. The Insertion Technique   Once the partner is comfortable, slowly insert one finger into the anal opening. Use a "come hither" motion to stimulate the rectal wall. This technique can be enhanced by:

- **Angle Adjustments:** Experiment with angles to find the most pleasurable spots, particularly the anterior wall where the prostate or G-spot may be located.
- **Rhythmic Movements:** Establish a rhythm that is comfortable for both partners, gradually increasing speed or pressure as desired.

3. The Two-Finger Technique   Once one finger is comfortably inserted, consider adding a second finger. This can provide a fuller sensation and allow for more varied stimulation. Position the fingers in a "V" shape to maximize contact with the internal walls.

4. The Curl and Press   For those looking to stimulate the prostate or G-spot, curl the fingers in a "come hither" motion while pressing against the front wall of the rectum. This technique can induce intense pleasure and lead to orgasm for many.

5. The Rotational Motion   Once comfortable with insertion, try rotating the fingers gently. This can create a unique sensation that enhances pleasure. Be mindful of the partner's responses and adjust accordingly.

Common Issues and Solutions

While finger techniques can be pleasurable, some challenges may arise:

- **Discomfort or Pain:** If the partner experiences discomfort, stop immediately. Ensure that adequate lubrication is used and that the partner is relaxed.
- **Difficulty with Insertion:** If insertion is challenging, increase foreplay and external stimulation. Consider using a smaller toy or finger first to ease into it.

- **Communication Breakdowns:** Maintain open lines of communication throughout the experience. If something feels off, check in with your partner and adjust as necessary.

Examples of Finger Techniques in Action

Solo Play: For those exploring anal play alone, fingers can be a great starting point. Begin by warming up the body with external stimulation, gradually introducing fingers into the anal area. Experiment with different techniques, such as the teasing touch or insertion technique, to discover what feels best.

Partner Play: When engaging with a partner, take turns exploring each other's bodies. Use the two-finger technique to stimulate the prostate or G-spot, while maintaining communication to ensure comfort and pleasure.

Conclusion

Finger techniques are an essential part of anal exploration, allowing individuals to connect with their bodies and their partners in new and exciting ways. Through understanding anatomy, preparation, and communication, finger play can lead to profound experiences of pleasure and intimacy. Embrace the journey, and remember that exploration is key to discovering what brings you and your partner joy.

External Stimulation

External stimulation refers to the pleasurable sensations experienced on the outside of the anal area, which can significantly enhance the overall enjoyment of anal play. This section will explore various techniques, theories, and practical applications of external stimulation, as well as address common challenges and considerations.

Theoretical Framework

The human body is a complex network of nerve endings, and the anal area is particularly rich in sensory receptors. Stimulation of these receptors can lead to heightened arousal and pleasure. Research indicates that external stimulation can activate the same neural pathways associated with orgasm, making it an essential component of anal pleasure.

The primary areas of focus for external stimulation include:

- The anal sphincters

- The perineum

- The surrounding skin

Each of these areas can be stimulated using various techniques, which we will explore in detail.

Techniques for External Stimulation

1. **Sphincter Stimulation** Lightly massaging the anal sphincters can create pleasurable sensations. Using a finger or a soft object, apply gentle pressure in circular motions. It's essential to communicate with your partner about the intensity and type of pressure that feels best.

2. **Perineum Massage** The perineum, located between the anus and the genitals, is another highly sensitive area. Applying pressure or using a vibrating toy on this area can enhance pleasure during anal play. Experiment with different techniques, such as tapping, rubbing, or using a rhythmic motion to discover what feels best.

3. **External Vibrators** Utilizing external vibrators can amplify sensations significantly. Placing a small, waterproof vibrator against the anus or perineum can provide thrilling vibrations that enhance arousal. Choose a toy with various settings to explore different levels of intensity.

4. **Temperature Play** Incorporating temperature into external stimulation can add an exciting dimension to anal play. Try using warm or cool objects, such as a warming lubricant or a chilled glass toy, to stimulate the anal area. Always ensure that the temperature is safe and comfortable to avoid any burns or discomfort.

5. **Feathers and Soft Materials** Using soft materials, such as feathers or silk, can create a tantalizing sensation on the sensitive skin around the anus. Lightly brushing these materials against the skin can build anticipation and heighten arousal.

Common Problems and Solutions

While external stimulation can be pleasurable, some individuals may experience discomfort or anxiety. Here are common challenges and practical solutions:

1. Discomfort from Pressure   If pressure on the anal area causes discomfort, it may be due to excessive force or inadequate relaxation. Ensure that both partners are relaxed and communicate openly about what feels good. Gradually increase pressure as comfort levels rise.

2. Anxiety and Tension   Anxiety can inhibit pleasure. To combat this, engage in relaxation techniques, such as deep breathing or gentle massaging of the body. Establishing a safe word can also help partners feel more secure during exploration.

3. Lack of Sensitivity   Some individuals may find they are less sensitive to external stimulation. Experimenting with different techniques, such as varying pressure, speed, and rhythm, can help identify what triggers pleasure. Additionally, ensuring that the area is well-lubricated can enhance sensitivity.

Examples of External Stimulation Scenarios

1. Partner Play   During partnered anal play, one partner can focus on stimulating the external areas while the other experiences internal sensations. This dual stimulation can create a powerful synergy, leading to intense pleasure.

2. Solo Exploration   For those exploring anal pleasure solo, external stimulation can be a great starting point. Use fingers or toys to explore the anal area, focusing on the sphincters and perineum. Experimenting with different techniques can help individuals discover their preferences.

3. Incorporating External Stimulation into Foreplay   External anal stimulation can be a thrilling addition to foreplay. It can heighten arousal before penetration, creating a more intense experience. Communicate with your partner about desires and preferences to enhance the experience.

Conclusion

External stimulation is a vital aspect of anal play that can significantly enhance pleasure. By understanding the anatomy, exploring various techniques, and addressing common challenges, individuals can unlock new levels of enjoyment. Remember, the key to successful external stimulation is open communication, consent, and a willingness to explore together. Embrace the journey of discovery and enjoy the pleasures that external stimulation can bring to your anal play experience.

Insertion and Exploration

When it comes to anal play, the act of insertion can be both exhilarating and intimidating. Understanding the body, the necessary preparations, and the techniques involved can transform the experience from a source of anxiety into one of profound pleasure. This section will delve into the intricacies of insertion and exploration, emphasizing the importance of safety, communication, and mindfulness.

The Importance of Patience

The first rule of anal insertion is patience. Rushing can lead to discomfort or pain, which can create negative associations with anal play. It is crucial to approach insertion with a mindset of exploration rather than a goal-oriented mindset. This means taking the time to listen to your body and your partner's body, allowing for gradual acclimatization to the sensations involved.

Preparing for Insertion

Before any insertion occurs, preparation is key. This involves both physical and mental readiness.

- **Hygiene:** Cleanliness is essential. Engaging in anal play should always be preceded by proper hygiene practices. This can include showering and using anal-specific cleansing products if desired.

- **Lubrication:** The anus does not self-lubricate, making lubrication a vital component of comfortable anal insertion. Use a high-quality, body-safe lubricant, preferably a water-based or silicone-based lubricant, as these provide the necessary slickness to ease insertion.

- **Relaxation:** Engaging in relaxation techniques such as deep breathing, gentle massage, or even a warm bath can help reduce tension in the anal sphincter, making insertion easier.

Techniques for Insertion

Once both partners are ready and comfortable, the following techniques can be employed for successful insertion:

1. Gradual Finger Insertion Begin with the use of fingers to familiarize the body with the sensation of anal play. Start with one finger, applying lubricant generously.

$$\text{Pressure} = \frac{\text{Force}}{\text{Area}} \quad \text{(Friction is minimized with adequate lubrication)} \quad (9)$$

Insert the finger slowly at an angle, allowing the anal sphincter to relax around it. Maintain open communication throughout the process, asking for feedback on comfort levels.

2. Use of Toys Anal toys, such as butt plugs or anal beads, can enhance the experience. When using toys, choose ones specifically designed for anal play, as they feature flared bases to prevent them from being lost inside the body.

- **Starting Small:** Begin with smaller toys and gradually increase size as comfort allows.

- **Vibrating Toys:** Consider incorporating vibrating toys, as they can provide additional stimulation and enhance the pleasure experience.

3. Partner Insertion If engaging in partnered play, the receiving partner should take an active role in guiding the insertion process. This can involve:

- **Positioning:** The receiving partner can control the angle and depth of insertion by adjusting their position. Positions such as lying on the side or being on hands and knees can provide greater control.

- **Breath Control:** Instruct the receiving partner to take deep breaths, exhaling slowly as insertion occurs. This helps to relax the body and ease the process.

Common Problems and Solutions

Despite the best preparations, challenges can arise during anal insertion. Here are some common issues and how to address them:

- **Discomfort or Pain:** If discomfort occurs, stop immediately. Assess the situation and consider using more lubricant or taking a break to relax. Communication is crucial; partners should express their feelings openly.

- **Tension in the Sphincter:** If the anal sphincter remains tense, it may be beneficial to return to external stimulation or use a smaller toy before attempting insertion again.
- **Loss of Control:** If the receiving partner feels overwhelmed, they should utilize a safe word or signal to pause or stop the activity. Establishing these beforehand is essential for a safe experience.

Exploration Beyond Insertion

Once insertion has been achieved, exploration can continue beyond simply pushing in and pulling out. The following techniques can enhance the experience:

- **Movement:** Experiment with different movements such as thrusting, rotating, or gentle wiggling to discover what feels best.
- **Depth Control:** Vary the depth of insertion to find the most pleasurable sensations. Some may enjoy shallow movements, while others may prefer deeper penetration.
- **Combining Stimulation:** For those with vaginas, combining anal play with vaginal stimulation (either through fingers or toys) can create a more intense experience.

Mindfulness and Presence

Throughout the process of insertion and exploration, maintaining mindfulness is crucial. This involves being fully present in the moment, focusing on the sensations, and being responsive to both your own and your partner's needs.

$$\text{Pleasure} = \text{Awareness} \times \text{Connection} \tag{10}$$

A heightened sense of awareness and connection can lead to deeper intimacy and satisfaction during anal play.

Conclusion

Insertion and exploration in anal play can be a deeply rewarding experience when approached with care, patience, and open communication. By understanding the body, preparing adequately, and employing mindful techniques, individuals and couples can unlock new realms of pleasure. Remember, the journey is as important as the destination—embrace the exploration and enjoy every moment of your anal adventure.

G-spot and Prostate Stimulation with Fingers

G-spot and prostate stimulation through finger techniques can lead to profound pleasure and heightened sexual experiences. Understanding the anatomy involved and employing the right techniques is crucial for maximizing pleasure and ensuring safety. This section will delve into the anatomy, techniques, and potential challenges associated with G-spot and prostate stimulation.

Anatomy Overview

G-spot Anatomy The G-spot, or Grafenberg spot, is located on the anterior wall of the vagina, approximately 1-3 inches inside the vaginal opening. It is often described as a spongy area that can swell when stimulated. Research suggests that the G-spot may be part of a larger network of erectile tissue that includes the clitoris and surrounding structures.

Prostate Anatomy The prostate gland is located about 2-3 inches inside the rectum, towards the front of the body. It is walnut-sized and can be stimulated through the rectal wall. The prostate is rich in nerve endings and can produce intense sensations when stimulated, often leading to powerful orgasms.

Techniques for Stimulation

G-spot Stimulation Techniques 1. **Positioning**: Ensure the receiver is comfortable and relaxed. Positions such as lying on their back with knees bent or in a doggy style position can facilitate access to the G-spot.
   2. **Finger Technique**:

- Insert one or two fingers into the vagina, curling them in a "come hither" motion towards the front wall.

- Apply varying pressure to find the G-spot. A gentle, rhythmic pressure is often most effective.

- Experiment with different angles and speeds to discover what feels best.

   3. **Combining Stimulation**:

BASIC ANAL TECHNIQUES 75

- Incorporate clitoral stimulation simultaneously for enhanced pleasure.
- Use a second hand to stimulate the clitoris or other erogenous zones.

Prostate Stimulation Techniques 1. **Preparation**: Ensure the receiver is relaxed and comfortable. Engaging in foreplay can help ease any tension.

2. **Finger Technique**:

- Insert one or two fingers into the rectum, aiming towards the belly button.
- Gently apply pressure to the prostate, using a "come hither" motion.
- Experiment with pressure and rhythm to find the most pleasurable sensations.

3. **Combining Stimulation**:

- For added pleasure, combine prostate stimulation with other forms of stimulation, such as anal or genital play.
- Consider using a vibrating toy alongside finger techniques for enhanced sensations.

Common Problems and Solutions

Discomfort or Pain If discomfort occurs during stimulation, it is essential to stop and reassess. Pain can be caused by insufficient lubrication, tension, or anxiety.

- **Solution**: Use plenty of water-based or silicone-based lubricant. Encourage relaxation and communication about what feels good or uncomfortable.

Difficulty Finding the G-spot or Prostate Some individuals may find it challenging to locate the G-spot or prostate initially.

- **Solution**: Experiment with different angles, positions, and levels of pressure. Use anatomical diagrams or descriptions to assist in locating these areas.

Emotional Barriers Some individuals may experience emotional barriers or anxiety related to anal or G-spot stimulation.

- **Solution**: Engage in open communication about desires, fears, and boundaries. Establish a safe word to ensure a comfortable experience.

Conclusion

G-spot and prostate stimulation with fingers can be an incredibly pleasurable experience when approached with care, knowledge, and communication. By understanding the anatomy involved and employing effective techniques, individuals can unlock new levels of pleasure and intimacy. Always prioritize consent, comfort, and safety to ensure a fulfilling exploration of these sensitive areas. Embrace the journey of discovery, and enjoy the pleasures that lie within.

Enhancing Pleasure with Different Finger Techniques

Anal play can be an incredibly pleasurable experience when approached with care and creativity. One of the most effective ways to enhance pleasure during anal exploration is through the use of various finger techniques. This section delves into the theory behind these techniques, common challenges, and practical examples to maximize pleasure during anal play.

Theoretical Foundations

The anus is rich in nerve endings, making it highly sensitive to touch. Understanding the anatomy of the anal area is crucial for maximizing pleasure. The external anal sphincter, located at the opening, is a muscular ring that can be stimulated directly. The internal structures, including the rectum and the surrounding tissues, also play a significant role in the overall experience.

$$\text{Pleasure} = f(\text{Nerve Endings}, \text{Technique}, \text{Consent}) \qquad (11)$$

This equation illustrates that pleasure is a function of the density of nerve endings, the technique employed, and the consent and comfort of all parties involved.

Common Problems and Solutions

While exploring anal play with fingers, individuals may encounter several challenges:

1. **Discomfort or Pain**: This can stem from insufficient lubrication, inadequate relaxation, or improper technique. Always prioritize communication and ensure that both partners feel comfortable.

2. **Lack of Sensation**: If the sensation is not as intense as expected, consider varying the speed, pressure, and angle of your finger movements.

3. **Difficulty in Relaxation**: Anxiety can inhibit relaxation, making anal play uncomfortable. Engage in foreplay and use relaxation techniques such as deep breathing or gentle massage to ease tension.

Techniques for Enhancing Pleasure

Here are several finger techniques that can amplify pleasure during anal play:

1. The Teasing Touch

Start with gentle exploration around the anal opening. Use the pads of your fingers to caress the skin, applying light pressure. This technique increases sensitivity and prepares the area for deeper stimulation.

1. Use one finger to circle around the anus in a slow, rhythmic motion.

2. Gradually increase pressure as your partner becomes more comfortable.

3. Incorporate varying speeds to keep the experience exciting.

2. The In-and-Out Motion

Once your partner is comfortable, introduce gentle insertion. This technique involves a rhythmic in-and-out motion that mimics penetration.

1. Start with a well-lubricated finger and slowly insert it into the anus.

2. Maintain a steady rhythm, pulling out slightly before pushing back in.

3. Adjust the angle to find the most pleasurable spots, such as the anterior wall, which is where the G-spot is located for some individuals.

3. The Curl and Press

This technique focuses on stimulating the internal structures, particularly the prostate in males and the G-spot in females.

1. Insert your finger and gently curl it towards the front of the body, applying pressure against the anterior wall.

2. Hold this position for a few seconds, allowing your partner to adjust to the sensation.

3. Experiment with different angles and pressures to discover what feels best.

4. The Scissor Technique

This technique involves using two fingers to create a scissor-like motion, which can provide a unique sensation.

1. Insert two fingers and position them in a scissor formation.

2. Gently open and close your fingers while maintaining contact with the anal walls.

3. This motion can create a pleasurable stretching sensation and enhance arousal.

5. The Finger Twist

The finger twist technique adds an element of rotation to the stimulation, which can enhance sensation.

1. Insert one or two fingers and gently rotate them in a circular motion.

2. Vary the speed and pressure to find the most pleasurable rhythm.

3. This technique can be particularly effective when combined with other movements, such as in-and-out or curling.

6. Combining Techniques

To maximize pleasure, consider combining different techniques. For example, you can alternate between the teasing touch and the curl and press to create a more dynamic experience. Communication is key—check in with your partner regularly to ensure they are enjoying the sensations.

Conclusion

Enhancing pleasure through different finger techniques can transform anal play into an exhilarating experience. By understanding the anatomy, addressing common challenges, and experimenting with various techniques, individuals can unlock new levels of pleasure. Remember, the key to a fulfilling experience lies in communication, consent, and creativity. Embrace the journey of exploration and enjoy the myriad sensations that anal play has to offer.

Toy Play

The world of anal play is vast and varied, and the introduction of toys can elevate your experience to new heights. Anal toys come in many shapes, sizes, and materials, allowing you to explore different sensations and techniques. This section will provide insights into choosing the right toys, techniques for solo and partner play, and safety considerations to ensure a pleasurable experience.

Choosing the Right Toys for Anal Play

When selecting anal toys, it is crucial to consider several factors to ensure safety and satisfaction. Here are some key points to keep in mind:

- **Material:** Anal toys should be made from non-porous materials such as silicone, glass, or stainless steel. These materials are easier to clean and less likely to harbor bacteria. Avoid porous materials like rubber or jelly, which can trap bacteria and cause infections.

- **Shape and Size:** Start with smaller toys if you are new to anal play. Gradually increase the size as you become more comfortable. Toys designed specifically for anal use often have flared bases to prevent them from getting lost inside the body.

- **Functionality:** Consider what sensations you wish to explore. Vibrating toys can add an exciting element to anal play, while non-vibrating toys can provide a different type of stimulation. Some toys are designed for dual use, stimulating both the anus and the vagina or prostate simultaneously.

- **Ease of Cleaning:** Ensure that the toys you choose are easy to clean. Look for toys that are waterproof or can be submerged in water for cleaning purposes. Always follow the manufacturer's instructions for cleaning and care.

Techniques for Solo Anal Play with Toys

Solo anal play can be a deeply satisfying experience. Here are some techniques to enhance your pleasure using anal toys:

1. **Preparation:** Before starting, ensure that you are in a comfortable and private space. Engage in relaxation techniques such as deep breathing or gentle stretching to prepare your body and mind for the experience.

2. **Lubrication:** Apply a generous amount of water-based or silicone-based lubricant to both the toy and your anal area. Lubrication is crucial for comfort and pleasure during anal play.

3. **Insertion:** Start by gently massaging the anal area with your fingers or the toy. Gradually introduce the toy, allowing your body to adjust to the sensation. Use slow, steady movements to avoid discomfort.

4. **Exploration:** Once the toy is inside, explore different angles and depths of penetration. Experiment with rocking, thrusting, or rotating the toy to discover what feels best for you. Pay attention to your body's responses and adjust accordingly.

5. **Vibration:** If using a vibrating toy, experiment with different settings and intensities. The added sensation can enhance your pleasure, especially when focused on sensitive areas such as the prostate or the anal walls.

Incorporating Toys into Partner Play

Anal toys can also enhance partnered experiences. Here are some tips for incorporating toys into your intimate encounters:

- **Communication:** Before introducing toys, discuss your desires and boundaries with your partner. Open communication is essential to ensure that both partners feel comfortable and excited about the experience.

- **Warm-Up:** Begin with foreplay to build arousal before introducing anal toys. This can include kissing, touching, or oral stimulation to heighten excitement.

- **Taking Turns:** Consider taking turns using the toy on each other. This can create a sense of shared pleasure and intimacy, allowing both partners to experience the sensations together.

- **Experimenting with Positions:** Certain positions may enhance the experience when using anal toys. For example, the receiving partner may find it pleasurable to be on their side or on all fours while the other partner uses the toy.

- **Aftercare:** After your session, take time for aftercare. This can include cuddling, discussing what you enjoyed, and cleaning the toys together. Aftercare helps to reinforce intimacy and connection between partners.

Safety Considerations

While anal toy play can be exhilarating, safety should always be a priority. Here are some essential safety tips:

- **Always Use Lubrication:** Anal play requires lubrication to prevent discomfort and injury. Never attempt anal play without sufficient lubricant.

- **Check for Damage:** Before using any toy, inspect it for damage or wear. Discontinue use if you notice any cracks, chips, or other signs of deterioration.

- **Use a Flared Base:** Ensure that any anal toy has a flared base to prevent it from becoming lost inside the body. This is especially important for toys designed for anal use.

- **Clean Before and After Use:** Always clean your toys before and after use to prevent infections. Use warm water and mild soap or a toy cleaner specifically designed for sexual toys.

- **Listen to Your Body:** Pay attention to your body's signals. If you experience pain or discomfort, stop immediately. Anal play should never be painful; if it is, reassess your technique and approach.

In conclusion, incorporating anal toys into your play can significantly enhance your pleasure and exploration. Whether you are engaging in solo play or sharing the experience with a partner, the right toys and techniques can lead to new and exciting sensations. Always prioritize safety and communication to ensure a fulfilling and enjoyable experience in your anal journey.

Choosing the Right Toys for Anal Play

When it comes to enhancing your anal experience, the right toys can make all the difference. Selecting anal toys requires careful consideration of various factors, including material, size, shape, and functionality. This section will guide you through the essential aspects of choosing the perfect anal toys to elevate your pleasure.

Material Matters

The first consideration when choosing anal toys is the material from which they are made. Different materials offer distinct sensations and levels of safety. Here are some common materials used in anal toys:

- **Silicone:** Body-safe, non-porous, and easy to clean, silicone is an excellent choice for anal toys. It provides a smooth texture that can enhance comfort during use.

- **Glass:** Glass toys are often used for their sleekness and ability to retain temperature. They can be heated or cooled for added stimulation. However, they require careful handling to avoid breakage.

- **Stainless Steel:** Like glass, stainless steel is non-porous and can be used for temperature play. Its weight can provide a unique sensation, but it should be used with caution to prevent discomfort.

- **Rubber and PVC:** These materials are often cheaper but can contain phthalates and other chemicals that may not be body-safe. Always check for body-safe labeling.

Size and Shape

The size and shape of anal toys are crucial for both comfort and pleasure. Beginners might want to start with smaller toys that are tapered for easier insertion. Here are some guidelines:

- **Beginners:** Start with toys that have a diameter of 1 inch (2.54 cm) or less. Tapered shapes are ideal for easing into anal play.

- **Intermediate Users:** Once comfortable, you can explore larger toys (1.5 inches or 3.81 cm in diameter) or those with unique shapes, such as curves designed to target the prostate or G-spot.

- **Advanced Users:** For those experienced in anal play, consider toys designed for advanced techniques, such as anal beads or large dildos. However, always prioritize safety and comfort.

Functionality and Design

Different toys serve different purposes, and understanding these can enhance your experience:

- **Dildos:** These come in various shapes and sizes, some designed for anal use with flared bases to prevent slipping. Consider a dildo with a curve for G-spot or prostate stimulation.

- **Vibrators:** Anal vibrators can provide additional stimulation. Look for ones specifically designed for anal use, with a flared base for safety.

- **Anal Beads:** These toys consist of a series of graduated beads that can provide a unique sensation during insertion and removal. They are excellent for those who enjoy the build-up of pleasure.

- **Prostate Massagers:** Specifically designed for prostate stimulation, these toys often have a curved shape to target the prostate effectively. Many also include vibration for added pleasure.

Safety Features

Safety should always be your top priority when choosing anal toys. Here are some essential safety features to look for:

- **Flared Base:** Ensure that any anal toy has a flared base to prevent the toy from being inserted too deeply, which can lead to complications.

- **Non-Porous Materials:** Opt for non-porous materials that can be easily sanitized. This reduces the risk of bacterial infections.

- **Easy to Clean:** Choose toys that can be cleaned with soap and water or are dishwasher-safe. Some materials can be boiled for sterilization.

Addressing Common Problems

While selecting the right toys, you may encounter common problems. Here are some solutions:

- **Discomfort during Use:** If you experience discomfort, it may be due to size or lack of lubrication. Always use a generous amount of water-based or silicone-based lubricant to enhance comfort.

- **Fear of Injury:** Take your time and listen to your body. If a toy feels too large or uncomfortable, stop and reassess. Gradual exploration is key to comfort and safety.

- **Cleaning Concerns:** Always clean your toys before and after use. Use warm water and mild soap, or a dedicated toy cleaner. For porous materials, consider using a condom over the toy to maintain hygiene.

Examples of Popular Anal Toys

To provide a clearer picture, here are a few examples of popular anal toys:

- **The Njoy Pure Wand:** Made from stainless steel, this toy is perfect for G-spot and prostate stimulation. Its weight and curvature provide intense pleasure.

- **Lelo Loki Wave:** This prostate massager features dual motors for internal and external stimulation, with a design that allows for comfortable use.

- **B-Vibe Rimming Plug:** This anal plug combines vibration with a unique rimming feature, offering a variety of sensations for advanced users.

Conclusion

Choosing the right anal toys can significantly enhance your pleasure and exploration. By considering materials, size, shape, functionality, and safety features, you can find toys that suit your needs and desires. Always prioritize communication with your partner and ensure that you are both comfortable with the toys you choose. Happy exploring!

Techniques for Solo Anal Play with Toys

Solo anal play can be an exhilarating and deeply satisfying experience, especially when incorporating toys designed specifically for anal stimulation. In this section, we will explore various techniques to enhance your solo play, ensuring safety, pleasure, and satisfaction.

Choosing the Right Toys

Selecting the appropriate toy is crucial for a pleasurable experience. Consider the following factors when choosing anal toys:

- **Size and Shape:** Start with smaller toys if you are a beginner. Gradually work your way up to larger sizes as you become more comfortable. Toys with flared bases are essential for safety, preventing the toy from getting lost inside.

- **Material:** Opt for body-safe materials such as silicone, glass, or stainless steel. These materials are non-porous and easy to clean, making them ideal for anal play.

- **Functionality:** Vibrating toys can add an extra layer of pleasure. Consider a toy that offers various settings to discover what feels best for you.

Preparation and Safety

Before diving into solo anal play, it's essential to prepare both physically and mentally.

- **Hygiene:** Ensure that both your body and your toys are clean. Wash your toys with warm water and mild soap or a toy cleaner.

- **Lubrication:** Use plenty of lubricant, as the anus does not produce its own lubrication. Silicone-based or water-based lubes are recommended. Apply liberally to both the toy and the anal area to minimize discomfort and enhance pleasure.

- **Relaxation:** Take time to relax your body and mind. Consider engaging in deep breathing exercises or a warm bath to ease tension.

Techniques for Solo Anal Play

Once you are prepared, you can begin exploring various techniques for solo anal play.

1. **External Stimulation** Start with external stimulation to help your body acclimate to anal play. Use your fingers or a small anal toy to gently massage the area around the anus. This can include:

    + **Circular Motions:** Use your fingers or a toy to make small circular motions around the anal opening, gradually increasing pressure as you become more comfortable.

    + **Pulsing:** Gently press the toy against the anus and release, creating a pulsing sensation that can heighten arousal.

2. **Insertion Techniques** Once you feel relaxed and aroused, you can begin to insert the toy.

    + **Gradual Insertion:** Start with the tip of the toy at the anal opening. Slowly and gently apply pressure, allowing your body to adjust to the sensation.

    + **Rocking Motion:** Once the tip is inside, use a gentle rocking motion to stimulate the anal walls and gradually push the toy deeper.

    + **Twisting:** If your toy allows for it, try twisting it slightly as you insert it. This can create unique sensations along the anal canal.

3. **Combining Techniques** For a more intense experience, combine different techniques:

    + **Vibration and Insertion:** If you're using a vibrating toy, turn it on before insertion. The vibrations can enhance the sensations as you insert the toy.

    + **G-Spot Stimulation:** If you are also exploring vaginal stimulation, consider using a curved toy that can stimulate both the anal and vaginal areas simultaneously.

    + **Breath Control:** Experiment with your breathing. Inhale deeply as you insert the toy and exhale as you push it deeper, syncing your breath with your movements for heightened pleasure.

4. **Experimenting with Angles and Positions** Changing your position can dramatically alter the sensations you experience during anal play:

- **Lying on Your Side:** This position can help you relax and allow for easier insertion.

- **On All Fours:** This position can create a more intense angle for deeper penetration and better access to the prostate for those with male anatomy.

- **Sitting:** Sitting on the toy can provide a unique sensation as you control the depth and angle of penetration.

5. **Aftercare** After your session, it's important to practice aftercare to ensure comfort and satisfaction:

- **Cleaning:** Wash your toys thoroughly after use. Clean yourself as well to maintain hygiene.

- **Reflection:** Take a moment to reflect on your experience. What felt good? What would you like to try next time? Journaling these thoughts can enhance your future sessions.

- **Relaxation:** Engage in a calming activity post-play, such as taking a warm shower or practicing mindfulness, to help you unwind.

Common Challenges

While exploring solo anal play, you may encounter some challenges:

- **Discomfort or Pain:** If you experience pain, stop immediately. Pain is a signal from your body that something is wrong. Reassess your technique, lubrication, and relaxation.

- **Difficulty with Insertion:** If you find insertion challenging, consider using a smaller toy first or focusing more on external stimulation before attempting penetration.

- **Mental Barriers:** If you feel anxiety or apprehension, take a step back. Explore your feelings and consider if you need more time to prepare mentally.

In conclusion, solo anal play with toys can be a rewarding and pleasurable experience when approached with care, preparation, and creativity. By understanding your body, choosing the right toys, and employing various techniques, you can unlock new realms of pleasure and satisfaction. Remember to prioritize safety, consent, and communication with yourself as you embark on this intimate journey.

Incorporating Toys into Partner Play

In the realm of anal play, incorporating toys can significantly enhance the experience for both partners. Toys not only add variety but also allow for exploration of new sensations, making the journey into anal pleasure more exciting and fulfilling. This section will delve into the practical aspects of integrating toys into partner play, addressing potential challenges, and providing examples to inspire creativity.

Choosing the Right Toys

When selecting toys for anal play with a partner, consider the following factors:

- **Material:** Choose body-safe materials such as silicone, glass, or stainless steel. These materials are non-porous and easy to clean, ensuring safety and hygiene.

- **Size and Shape:** Start with smaller toys if either partner is new to anal play. Consider the shape of the toy; curved designs can target the prostate or G-spot effectively.

- **Functionality:** Vibrating toys can provide additional stimulation, while non-vibrating options can be used for more traditional anal penetration. Consider the dynamics of your play and choose toys that complement your desires.

Communication is Key

Before incorporating toys into partner play, open communication is essential. Discuss preferences, boundaries, and any concerns regarding the use of toys. Establishing a safe word or signal can help both partners feel secure and respected throughout the experience.

Techniques for Incorporating Toys

Here are some techniques to seamlessly introduce toys into partner play:

1. **Warm-Up with Fingers:** Begin with fingers to help relax the anal muscles and provide a sense of comfort. Gradually introduce the toy once both partners feel ready.

2. **Use Toys During Foreplay:** Incorporate toys during foreplay to heighten arousal. For example, use a small anal plug while engaging in oral or vaginal stimulation.

3. **Take Turns:** Allow each partner to take turns using the toy. This can create a sense of anticipation and excitement, as each partner experiences pleasure in different ways.

4. **Combine with Other Forms of Stimulation:** Use toys in conjunction with other forms of stimulation, such as oral sex or manual stimulation, to create a multi-layered experience. For instance, a partner could use a vibrator on their own body while the other penetrates with a toy.

5. **Experiment with Positions:** Different positions can change how the toy feels during penetration. Try positions such as doggy style, missionary, or side-by-side to discover what feels best for both partners.

Addressing Potential Challenges

While incorporating toys can enhance the experience, it may also present challenges. Here are some common issues and solutions:

- **Discomfort:** If either partner feels discomfort, it's crucial to stop and reassess. Ensure that adequate lubrication is used and that the toy is the appropriate size and shape for both partners.

- **Loss of Connection:** Sometimes, the focus on the toy can detract from the emotional connection between partners. To combat this, maintain eye contact, engage in verbal affirmations, and ensure that both partners are actively participating in the experience.

- **Cleaning and Hygiene:** Ensure that toys are cleaned thoroughly before and after use. Discuss hygiene practices openly to ensure comfort and safety for both partners.

Examples of Toy Integration

Here are a few scenarios to illustrate how toys can be effectively integrated into partner play:

- **Vibrating Anal Plug:** One partner can wear a vibrating anal plug during intercourse. The vibrations can enhance pleasure for both partners, while the plug provides additional stimulation to the anal area.

- **Double Penetration with Toys:** Use a dildo or another penetrative toy alongside anal penetration. This can create a sense of fullness and enhance pleasure for both partners.

- **Using a Remote-Controlled Toy:** One partner can control a remote-controlled anal toy while the other engages in different forms of stimulation. This adds an element of surprise and excitement to the experience.

Conclusion

Incorporating toys into partner play can elevate the experience of anal pleasure, allowing for exploration, excitement, and deeper connection. By choosing the right toys, communicating openly, and experimenting with different techniques, partners can create memorable and fulfilling experiences together. Remember, the key is to prioritize safety, comfort, and consent, ensuring that both partners feel empowered and excited to explore the world of anal play together.

Advanced Toy Techniques for Intense Pleasure

When it comes to anal play, the right toys can elevate your experience from pleasurable to mind-blowing. In this section, we will explore advanced techniques for using anal toys effectively, ensuring that you maximize your pleasure while prioritizing safety and comfort.

Choosing the Right Toys

The first step in enhancing your anal play is selecting the appropriate toys. Consider the following factors:

- **Material:** Opt for body-safe materials such as silicone, glass, or stainless steel. Each material offers a different sensation; silicone is soft and flexible,

BASIC ANAL TECHNIQUES

while glass and stainless steel provide firmness and can be heated or cooled for temperature play.

- **Size and Shape:** Start with toys that are tapered or have a flared base to prevent any mishaps. As you become more comfortable, you can experiment with larger sizes or unique shapes designed to stimulate the prostate or G-spot.

- **Vibration:** Many anal toys come with vibration settings. Consider whether you want a toy that vibrates, as this can enhance sensations significantly.

Techniques for Solo Anal Play with Toys

When using toys for solo anal play, follow these techniques to maximize pleasure:

1. **Warm-Up:** Begin with gentle external stimulation. Use your fingers or a small external toy to stimulate the perineum and surrounding areas to relax the muscles and prepare for insertion.

2. **Gradual Insertion:** Slowly insert the toy, allowing your body to adjust to the sensation. Use plenty of lubricant to facilitate smooth entry.

3. **Movement:** Once inserted, experiment with different movements. Try gentle thrusting, twisting, or vibrating the toy to discover what feels best for you.

4. **Breathing Techniques:** Incorporate deep breathing to help relax your body. Inhale deeply through your nose, hold for a moment, and exhale slowly through your mouth. This can enhance relaxation and pleasure.

Incorporating Toys into Partner Play

When introducing toys into partner play, communication and consent are vital. Here are some techniques:

- **Discuss Desires:** Before play, have an open discussion with your partner about what you both want to explore. This includes the type of toys you wish to use and any boundaries you may have.

- **Take Turns:** Consider taking turns using the toy on each other. This creates a shared experience that can enhance intimacy and connection.

- **Use Toys for Stimulation:** While engaging in penetrative anal sex, one partner can use a toy to stimulate the G-spot or prostate simultaneously. This can be done with a vibrating toy or a double-ended dildo.

Advanced Techniques for Intense Pleasure

For those looking to push their boundaries, consider the following advanced techniques:

1. **Temperature Play:** Experiment with temperature by using glass or metal toys. Soak them in warm water or place them in the refrigerator for a few minutes before use. The contrasting sensations can heighten arousal.

2. **Anal Training:** Gradually increase the size of the toys you use. Start with smaller toys and work your way up to larger ones. This not only enhances pleasure but also helps your body adjust to different sizes.

3. **Combining Toys:** Use multiple toys simultaneously for a layered experience. For example, you can insert a vibrating anal plug while using a dildo for vaginal penetration, enhancing sensations for both partners.

4. **Mindful Focus:** During play, focus on the sensations in your body. Try to remain present and aware of how each movement and sensation affects you. This mindfulness can lead to deeper pleasure and satisfaction.

Common Problems and Solutions

While using anal toys, you may encounter some common issues. Here are solutions to help you navigate these challenges:

- **Discomfort or Pain:** If you experience discomfort, stop immediately. Reassess your technique, ensure you're using enough lubricant, and consider using a smaller toy. Never push through pain.

- **Difficulty with Insertion:** If you're having trouble with insertion, focus on relaxation techniques, such as deep breathing or gentle massage. A warm bath can also help relax your muscles before play.

- **Loss of Interest:** If you find your interest waning, change up the routine. Try different toys, positions, or incorporate roleplay to reignite excitement.

Conclusion

Advanced toy techniques can significantly enhance your anal play experience, leading to intense pleasure and deeper connections with your partner. Remember to prioritize safety, consent, and communication throughout your exploration. By experimenting with different toys and techniques, you can unlock new realms of pleasure, embracing the full spectrum of your desires.

Advanced Anal Techniques

Double Penetration

Double penetration (DP) is an exhilarating sexual practice that involves simultaneous penetration of the anus and vagina or anus and penis. This technique can amplify pleasure and create intense sensations, but it requires careful consideration of anatomy, communication, and safety.

Understanding Double Penetration

Double penetration can be experienced in various ways, whether through the use of two partners or the incorporation of toys alongside a partner. The essence of DP lies in the heightened stimulation that occurs when multiple erogenous zones are engaged at once.

$$\text{Total Pleasure} = \text{Pleasure from Penetration 1} + \text{Pleasure from Penetration 2} \tag{12}$$

This equation illustrates that the total pleasure experienced during double penetration is the sum of the pleasures derived from each penetration. However, the experience can vary significantly based on individual preferences, comfort levels, and the dynamics between partners.

Techniques for Double Penetration

1. **Positioning** Choosing the right position is crucial for a successful double penetration experience. Some popular positions include:

   - **Doggy Style:** The receiving partner is on all fours, allowing for easy access to both the vagina and anus.
   - **Spooning:** Partners lie on their sides, with the receiving partner's back against the penetrating partner's front, allowing for a more intimate experience.
   - **Cowgirl:** The receiving partner straddles one partner while the other penetrates from behind, allowing for control over depth and angle.

2. Communication   Before engaging in double penetration, it is imperative to have open discussions about desires, boundaries, and safe words. Establishing a safe word ensures that all parties can communicate their comfort levels effectively.

Challenges and Tips for Successful Double Penetration

Engaging in double penetration can present challenges, particularly concerning comfort and coordination between partners. Here are some tips to navigate these challenges:

- **Start Slow:** Gradually introduce penetration, allowing the receiving partner to acclimate to the sensations.

- **Use Plenty of Lubrication:** Adequate lubrication is essential to ensure comfort and ease of penetration. Silicone-based lubricants are often recommended for anal play due to their long-lasting properties.

- **Focus on Breathing:** Encourage the receiving partner to focus on their breathing to help relax the muscles and enhance pleasure.

- **Check In Regularly:** Continuous communication during the act is vital. Partners should frequently check in with each other to ensure comfort and pleasure.

Safety Precautions

Safety is paramount when exploring double penetration. Here are key precautions to consider:

- **Use Condoms:** If engaging in double penetration with two partners, using condoms can reduce the risk of sexually transmitted infections (STIs).

- **Hygiene Practices:** Ensure that all toys and body parts are clean before and after use to prevent infections.

- **Listen to Your Body:** If any discomfort or pain arises, it is essential to stop immediately. Pain is a signal that something may be wrong.

Exploring Fantasies and Desires

Double penetration can also be an avenue to explore fantasies and desires. Partners may wish to incorporate elements of roleplay or power dynamics into their DP experience. Discussing these fantasies openly can enhance intimacy and create a more fulfilling experience.

Conclusion

Double penetration can be a thrilling and pleasurable experience when approached with care, communication, and consent. By understanding the anatomy involved, employing effective techniques, and prioritizing safety, partners can unlock the full potential of this exhilarating practice. Embrace the journey of exploration, and let the pleasures of double penetration enhance your sexual repertoire.

Diverse Options for Double Penetration

Double penetration (DP) is an exhilarating experience that can amplify pleasure and connection between partners. This section explores the diverse options available for engaging in double penetration, considering various techniques, positions, and considerations to enhance safety and pleasure.

Understanding Double Penetration

Double penetration typically involves simultaneous penetration of two orifices, most commonly the vagina and anus. This practice can be achieved with different combinations of partners and body parts, including:

- Two partners using their bodies (e.g., one partner penetrating the vagina while the other penetrates the anus).
- A single partner using a toy or appendage for one orifice while the other is penetrated by another partner.
- Utilizing sex toys designed for double penetration, such as dual-ended dildos or specialized anal/vaginal toys.

Positions for Double Penetration

Choosing the right position is crucial for comfort and pleasure during double penetration. Here are some popular positions that facilitate DP:

- **Missionary with a Twist**: The receiving partner lies on their back with legs raised, while one partner penetrates the vagina and the other penetrates the anus from a kneeling position. This position allows for face-to-face intimacy and easy communication.

- **Doggy Style**: The receiving partner is on all fours, allowing one partner to penetrate the anus from behind while the other penetrates the vagina from below. This position provides deep penetration and can be adjusted for comfort.

- **Spooning**: Partners lie side by side, with one partner penetrating the vagina and the other the anus. This position offers a sense of closeness and intimacy while allowing for gentle penetration.

- **The Bridge**: The receiving partner lies on their back and lifts their hips, supported by their shoulders and feet, creating a bridge-like position. One partner can penetrate the vagina while the other penetrates the anus. This position allows for a unique angle of penetration.

- **Cowgirl with Support**: The receiving partner straddles one partner while facing them, allowing them to control the depth and angle of vaginal penetration. The other partner can penetrate the anus from behind, providing simultaneous stimulation.

Techniques for Successful Double Penetration

To ensure a pleasurable experience, consider the following techniques:

- **Communication**: Open dialogue is essential. Discuss boundaries, desires, and comfort levels before engaging in double penetration. Establish safe words and signals to ensure everyone feels secure and respected.

- **Gradual Insertion**: Start slowly to allow the receiving partner to adjust to the sensations. Gradual insertion helps prevent discomfort and allows for increased arousal.

- **Use of Lubrication**: Adequate lubrication is crucial for comfort during double penetration. Use high-quality water-based or silicone-based lubricants to enhance the experience. Reapply as needed to maintain smoothness.

- **Pacing:** Maintain a comfortable pace that accommodates the receiving partner's comfort level. Encourage feedback to adjust speed and depth as needed.

- **Alternate Rhythms:** Partners can synchronize their movements or alternate rhythms to create varied sensations. This can enhance the overall experience and keep it exciting.

Challenges and Considerations

While double penetration can be immensely pleasurable, it also comes with potential challenges:

- **Physical Discomfort:** Some may experience discomfort during DP, particularly if they are new to anal play. It is essential to listen to the body and communicate openly about any discomfort.

- **Anatomical Limitations:** Not all bodies are suited for double penetration. Individual anatomy and comfort levels vary, and it is crucial to respect personal boundaries.

- **Safety Concerns:** Always prioritize safety. Use condoms on toys and partners to minimize the risk of infection. Ensure that all participants are comfortable and consenting.

- **Emotional Considerations:** Engaging in DP can evoke various emotions. It is vital to check in with each other before, during, and after the experience to ensure everyone feels safe and respected.

Conclusion

Double penetration offers a unique opportunity for exploration and pleasure. By understanding diverse options, employing effective techniques, and addressing challenges, partners can create a fulfilling and enjoyable experience. Remember, communication and consent are key to unlocking the full potential of double penetration, leading to deeper intimacy and satisfaction.

$$\text{Pleasure} = \text{Communication} + \text{Consent} + \text{Technique} + \text{Exploration} \qquad (13)$$

Positions and Techniques for Simultaneous Pleasure

In the realm of anal play, the quest for simultaneous pleasure is an exhilarating journey that can enhance intimacy and satisfaction for all parties involved. This section explores various positions and techniques that facilitate dual stimulation, ensuring that both partners can enjoy the experience to its fullest.

Understanding Simultaneous Pleasure

Simultaneous pleasure in anal play refers to the ability to engage in activities that provide pleasure to both partners at the same time. This can involve a combination of anal penetration, vaginal stimulation, and other forms of sexual engagement. The essence of achieving simultaneous pleasure lies in the connection between partners, communication, and the right positioning.

Key Considerations

Before diving into specific positions, consider the following factors that can impact the experience:

- **Comfort and Flexibility:** Both partners should feel comfortable in the chosen position. Flexibility can enhance the experience, allowing for adjustments as needed.
- **Communication:** Open dialogue about desires, boundaries, and comfort levels is crucial. Establish safe words and signals to ensure a positive experience.
- **Anatomical Awareness:** Understanding each other's anatomy can help in selecting positions that maximize pleasure. Familiarize yourself with key erogenous zones, such as the G-spot and the prostate.
- **Lubrication:** Adequate lubrication is essential for anal play to prevent discomfort and enhance pleasure. Use high-quality water-based or silicone-based lubricants.

Positions for Simultaneous Pleasure

1. The Spooning Position

In this intimate position, both partners lie on their sides, with the receiving partner's back against the front of the penetrating partner. This position allows for close body contact, facilitating warmth and intimacy. The penetrating partner can easily access the anal area while the receiving partner can enjoy stimulation of the clitoris or other erogenous zones.

$$\text{Pleasure} = \text{Intimacy} + \text{Comfort} + \text{Accessibility} \qquad (14)$$

The spooning position is particularly beneficial for those new to anal play, as it provides a sense of security and control.

2. The Cowgirl Position

The receiving partner straddles the penetrating partner in this position, allowing them to control the depth and angle of penetration. This position not only empowers the receiving partner but also enables them to stimulate their own clitoris or engage in breast play, enhancing pleasure for both.

$$\text{Control} = \frac{\text{Depth} + \text{Angle}}{\text{Trust}} \qquad (15)$$

The cowgirl position is ideal for exploring different rhythms and movements, making it a favorite among many couples.

3. The Doggy Style Position

In this classic position, the receiving partner is on all fours while the penetrating partner enters from behind. This position allows for deep penetration and can be combined with clitoral stimulation from the penetrating partner's hands or a toy.

$$\text{Intensity} = \text{Depth of Penetration} \times \text{Clitoral Stimulation} \qquad (16)$$

Doggy style can also facilitate more adventurous elements, such as light spanking or impact play, adding layers to the experience.

4. The Face-to-Face Position

This position involves both partners sitting facing each other, with the receiving partner on the penetrating partner's lap. This intimate position allows for eye contact and kissing, creating a deep emotional connection while facilitating anal penetration.

$$\text{Connection} = \text{Eye Contact} + \text{Kissing} + \text{Penetration} \qquad (17)$$

The face-to-face position can also be adapted for additional stimulation, such as using a toy or fingers for clitoral or prostate stimulation.

5. The Side-By-Side Position

Both partners lie on their sides facing each other, with the penetrating partner positioned behind the receiving partner. This position allows for gentle penetration and easy access to clitoral stimulation, promoting a sense of closeness.

$$\text{Pleasure} = \text{Gentleness} + \text{Access to Erogenous Zones} \qquad (18)$$

The side-by-side position is excellent for extended sessions, as it allows for relaxation and continuous exploration.

Techniques for Enhancing Simultaneous Pleasure

To maximize the pleasure derived from the aforementioned positions, consider incorporating the following techniques:

- **Varying Speed and Rhythm:** Experiment with different speeds and rhythms during penetration. Slow, deliberate movements can build anticipation, while faster thrusts can increase intensity.

- **Incorporating Toys:** Use anal beads, vibrators, or other toys to enhance stimulation. Toys can be used on the receiving partner during penetration or vice versa.

- **Breath Play:** Synchronizing breathing can enhance the connection between partners. Try inhaling and exhaling together to create a rhythm that matches the movements.

- **Verbal Communication:** Encourage each other with words of affirmation and guidance. Express what feels good and what could be adjusted for more pleasure.

Common Challenges and Solutions

While exploring simultaneous pleasure, couples may encounter challenges such as discomfort, miscommunication, or difficulty finding the right rhythm. Here are some common problems and suggested solutions:

1. **Discomfort:** If either partner experiences discomfort, it's crucial to stop and reassess. Adjust positions, increase lubrication, or take a break if necessary.

2. **Miscommunication:** Establish clear communication protocols before engaging in anal play. Use safe words and signals to ensure both partners feel comfortable expressing their needs.

3. **Difficulty Finding Rhythm:** If you struggle to find a rhythm, try switching positions or taking turns being in control. Experimenting with different techniques can help both partners find their groove.

Conclusion

Achieving simultaneous pleasure in anal play is an art that requires exploration, communication, and a willingness to experiment. By understanding the anatomy, selecting the right positions, and employing effective techniques, couples can unlock a world of shared pleasure. Remember that the journey is just as important as the destination; embrace the experience, celebrate your connection, and enjoy every moment of your anal adventure.

Challenges and Tips for Successful Double Penetration

Double penetration (DP) can be an exhilarating and intensely pleasurable experience, but it also comes with its unique set of challenges. Understanding these challenges and employing effective strategies can help ensure a safe, enjoyable, and fulfilling experience for all parties involved.

Understanding the Challenges

1. Physical Comfort: One of the primary challenges with double penetration is ensuring physical comfort. The body has its limits, and pushing beyond them can lead to discomfort or pain. It is vital to communicate openly about comfort levels and to start slowly, allowing the body to adjust to the sensations of simultaneous penetration.

2. Coordination: Successful double penetration requires a degree of coordination between partners. This can be especially challenging if the partners are not familiar with each other's movements or if there is a significant difference in size between the two penetrative objects (e.g., a penis and a toy). Practicing synchronization and communication can mitigate this challenge.

3. Emotional Readiness: Engaging in double penetration can evoke a range of emotions, from excitement to anxiety. It is crucial for all participants to feel emotionally prepared and to have established trust and intimacy. Discussing fantasies, desires, and any fears beforehand can help create a supportive environment.

4. Safety Concerns: Safety is paramount in any sexual activity, especially in double penetration. It is essential to consider the use of condoms to prevent the transmission of sexually transmitted infections (STIs) and to ensure proper hygiene practices to avoid infections. Discussing boundaries and establishing safe words can also enhance safety.

Tips for Successful Double Penetration

1. Start with Foreplay: Engaging in extensive foreplay can help relax the body and increase arousal, making it easier to accommodate both penetrative objects. Focus on stimulating erogenous zones, utilizing fingers or toys, and building anticipation.

2. Use Plenty of Lubrication: Lubrication is crucial for enhancing comfort during double penetration. Opt for a high-quality lubricant that is suitable for the type of penetration involved (water-based for toys, silicone-based for anal). Apply generously to both the penetrative objects and the receiving partner.

3. Choose the Right Positions: Experimenting with different positions can help find what works best for everyone involved. Some popular positions for double penetration include:

- **Doggy Style:** This position allows for deep penetration and easy access for both partners.
- **Missionary with Legs Raised:** The receiving partner can lie on their back with legs raised, allowing for penetration from both angles.
- **Spooning:** This position offers intimacy and allows for controlled penetration, making it easier to communicate and adjust as needed.

4. Communicate Constantly: Communication is key to a successful double penetration experience. Partners should express their comfort levels, desires, and any discomfort that arises. Establishing a safe word can provide a clear signal to stop if needed.

5. Take It Slow: Rushing into double penetration can lead to discomfort or anxiety. Start with one penetrative object and gradually introduce the second. Allow time for the body to adjust to each penetration, and encourage the receiving partner to guide the pace.

ADVANCED ANAL TECHNIQUES

6. Focus on Pleasure: Remember that the goal of double penetration is pleasure for all involved. Pay attention to each other's reactions and adjust techniques accordingly. Consider incorporating other forms of stimulation, such as clitoral or nipple stimulation, to enhance the experience.

7. Aftercare: Aftercare is an essential component of any intense sexual experience. After engaging in double penetration, take time to cuddle, talk, and check in with each other emotionally and physically. This can strengthen the bond between partners and promote a positive experience.

Conclusion

Double penetration can be a thrilling addition to one's sexual repertoire, offering unique sensations and heightened pleasure. By understanding the challenges and employing effective strategies, partners can create a safe, enjoyable, and fulfilling experience. Remember, the essence of any sexual exploration lies in trust, communication, and mutual respect. Embrace the journey, and enjoy the exploration of pleasure together.

Anal Fisting

Anal fisting is an advanced sexual technique that involves the insertion of a hand, typically with one or more fingers extended, into the anus. This practice can yield intense sensations and create profound feelings of intimacy and trust between partners. However, it requires careful preparation, communication, and an understanding of anatomy to ensure safety and pleasure.

Understanding Anatomy and Safety Precautions

Before engaging in anal fisting, it is crucial to have a solid understanding of the anatomy involved. The anal canal is approximately **3 to 4 inches** long and is surrounded by sphincter muscles that can be trained to relax and accommodate larger objects. The rectum can stretch significantly, but it is vital to approach this practice with care to avoid injury.

Safety Precautions:

- **Hygiene:** Ensure that both partners practice good hygiene. Washing hands and trimming nails can prevent infections and discomfort.

- **Lubrication:** Use a generous amount of lubricant, as the anus does not produce natural lubrication. Silicone-based or water-based lubricants are recommended for this purpose.

- **Communication:** Establish a safe word or signal that either partner can use to pause or stop the activity at any time. This is crucial for maintaining trust and ensuring comfort.

- **Gradual Progression:** Start with fingers before progressing to the entire hand. This allows the receiving partner to adjust to the sensation and reduces the risk of injury.

Techniques for Gradual and Sensational Fisting

Fisting should always be approached with patience and care. Here are some techniques to facilitate a pleasurable experience:

1. **Warm-Up:** Begin with gentle anal play to relax the sphincter muscles. Use one or two fingers to stimulate the anus and surrounding areas. Gradually increase pressure and depth as comfort allows.

2. **Finger Techniques:** Once the partner is adequately warmed up, explore different finger techniques. For instance, curling the fingers in a "come hither" motion can stimulate the rectal wall and enhance pleasure.

3. **Gradual Insertion:** When the receiving partner feels ready, slowly insert the hand. Start with one finger, then two, and gradually work up to the entire hand. Ensure that the partner is comfortable and responsive throughout the process.

4. **Positioning:** Experiment with different positions to find what feels best. Some may prefer lying on their side, while others may find it more comfortable to be on their hands and knees.

5. **Breathing Techniques:** Encourage deep, steady breathing. This can help relax the body and ease any tension, making the experience more enjoyable.

Communication and Trust during Fisting

Engaging in anal fisting requires a high level of trust between partners. It is essential to maintain open lines of communication throughout the experience. Here are some strategies to enhance communication and trust:

- **Check-Ins:** Regularly check in with your partner about their comfort level. Simple questions like, "How does that feel?" or "Do you want to go slower?" can make a significant difference.

- **Encourage Feedback:** Encourage your partner to express their feelings and desires. This can help tailor the experience to their preferences and enhance pleasure.

- **Aftercare:** After the session, engage in aftercare to help your partner feel safe and cared for. This can include cuddling, discussing the experience, or simply being present together.

Exploring Power Dynamics with Anal Fisting

For some, anal fisting can also be a way to explore power dynamics within a relationship. This can involve elements of dominance and submission, which can heighten the experience. Here are some considerations:

- **Consent:** Always ensure that consent is enthusiastic and ongoing. Discuss boundaries and desires before engaging in any power exchange activities.

- **Roleplay:** Incorporate roleplay scenarios to enhance the experience. This can involve one partner taking on a more dominant role while the other submits to the experience.

- **Control:** The dominant partner can control the pace and depth of penetration, while the submissive partner can focus on surrendering to the sensations.

Conclusion

Anal fisting can be an incredibly pleasurable and intimate experience when approached with care, communication, and consent. By understanding the anatomy involved, practicing safety precautions, and fostering trust between partners, individuals can explore this advanced technique in a way that enhances their sexual journey. Remember to take your time, listen to your partner, and enjoy the exploration of pleasure together.

Understanding Anatomy and Safety Precautions

Understanding the anatomy involved in anal play is crucial for maximizing pleasure and minimizing risks. This section will explore the relevant anatomical structures, the importance of safety precautions, and the potential problems that can arise during anal activities.

Anatomical Overview

The anal area consists of several key components that play a significant role in pleasure and sensation:

- **The Anus:** The external opening of the rectum, surrounded by the anal sphincter muscles, which control the passage of stool and can also provide pleasurable sensations when stimulated.
- **Rectum:** The part of the large intestine that connects the anus to the sigmoid colon. It is approximately 12 centimeters long and is highly sensitive due to the presence of nerve endings.
- **Sphincter Muscles:** These muscles consist of two main components: the internal anal sphincter, which is involuntary, and the external anal sphincter, which is under voluntary control. Understanding how to relax these muscles is essential for comfortable anal play.
- **Perineum:** The area between the anus and the genitals, rich in nerve endings, and can be stimulated to enhance pleasure during anal activities.

Safety Precautions

Engaging in anal play requires careful consideration of safety to prevent injury and ensure a pleasurable experience. Here are key safety precautions to keep in mind:

- **Consent and Communication:** Prior to any anal play, it is essential to have open discussions with your partner about desires, boundaries, and consent. Establishing a safe word or signal can facilitate communication during the act.
- **Hygiene:** Cleanliness is vital to prevent infections. Consider using an enema before anal play, though this should be done cautiously and not excessively. Always wash hands and any toys before and after use.
- **Lubrication:** The anus does not self-lubricate, so using a generous amount of lubricant is necessary to prevent friction and discomfort. Water-based or silicone-based lubricants are recommended, as oil-based products can degrade latex condoms.
- **Gradual Insertion:** Begin with gentle, slow movements to allow the body to adjust. Start with fingers or small toys before progressing to larger items. Listening to your body and your partner's cues is crucial.

- **Using Protection:** If engaging in anal sex, consider using condoms to reduce the risk of sexually transmitted infections (STIs). Change condoms between anal and vaginal intercourse to prevent bacterial transfer.

- **Recognizing Pain:** Distinguish between discomfort and pain. If pain occurs, stop immediately and reassess the situation. Pain can indicate that something is wrong, such as excessive force or insufficient lubrication.

Potential Problems

Despite the pleasures associated with anal play, several issues can arise if safety precautions are not followed:

- **Tears and Fissures:** The delicate skin of the anal area can tear if not properly prepared. This can lead to painful fissures, which may require medical attention.

- **Infections:** Poor hygiene can lead to bacterial infections. Symptoms may include unusual discharge, itching, or discomfort. Seek medical advice if these symptoms occur.

- **Psychological Effects:** Emotional responses to anal play can vary. Some may feel pleasure, while others may experience anxiety or discomfort. It is important to address these feelings and communicate openly with your partner.

- **Physical Discomfort:** Some individuals may experience physical discomfort during anal play due to tightness or lack of relaxation. Techniques such as deep breathing and gradual insertion can help alleviate this issue.

Conclusion

Understanding the anatomy involved in anal play, along with adhering to safety precautions, is essential for a fulfilling and pleasurable experience. By communicating openly, prioritizing hygiene, using lubrication, and recognizing the body's signals, you can explore anal play safely and enjoyably. Always remember that pleasure should never come at the cost of safety, and taking the time to prepare can lead to more satisfying experiences.

Techniques for Gradual and Sensational Fisting

Fisting can be an incredibly intimate and pleasurable experience when approached with care, patience, and an understanding of anatomy. This section will explore techniques for gradual and sensational fisting, emphasizing the importance of communication, preparation, and listening to your partner's body.

Understanding the Anatomy

Before engaging in fisting, it's crucial to understand the anatomy involved. The anal canal is typically about 3 to 4 inches long, with the rectum extending further into the body. The goal of fisting is to stretch the anal sphincter and the surrounding muscles gradually. This requires a deep understanding of the body's limits and the ability to read physical cues.

Preparation

- **Mental Preparation:** Both partners should be mentally prepared for the experience. Discuss desires, boundaries, and any fears or concerns beforehand. This builds trust and ensures a more enjoyable experience.
- **Physical Preparation:** Engage in a thorough warm-up routine. This can include anal stretching with fingers or small toys, as well as relaxation techniques to ease any tension in the body.
- **Hygiene:** Cleanliness is paramount in anal play. Consider an enema if desired, but ensure that it's done safely and comfortably.

Gradual Insertion Techniques

1. **Start Small:** Begin with one or two fingers. Use plenty of water-based or silicone-based lubricant to ensure comfort. Gradually work your way up to three fingers, allowing the body to adjust.
2. **Pulsing Motion:** Once you have three fingers comfortably inside, use a gentle pulsing motion. This rhythmic movement can help relax the anal sphincter and prepare it for more significant stretching.
3. **Slow and Steady:** When transitioning to the fist, it's critical to maintain a slow pace. The fist should be angled slightly, with the thumb positioned either alongside the fingers or tucked in, creating a more comfortable shape for insertion.

4. **Listening to the Body:** Pay close attention to your partner's verbal and non-verbal cues. If they express discomfort, slow down or take a break. Communication is key to ensuring safety and pleasure.

Sensational Techniques

Fisting is not just about the act itself but also about creating sensations that enhance pleasure. Here are techniques to explore:

- **Pressure Points:** As the fist is inserted, gently press against the walls of the rectum. This can stimulate sensitive areas, including the prostate in males and the anterior wall in females, creating intense sensations.

- **Twisting and Curling:** Once fully inserted, experiment with twisting the fist or curling the fingers. This movement can create different sensations and stimulate various nerve endings.

- **Varying Depth:** Play with depth by withdrawing slightly and then pushing back in. This can create a rhythmic sensation that heightens arousal.

- **Breath Control:** Encourage your partner to control their breathing. Deep, slow breaths can help them relax and enhance the sensations experienced during fisting.

Common Challenges

Engaging in fisting can present challenges. Here are some common issues and solutions:

- **Discomfort or Pain:** If discomfort arises, stop immediately. Pain is a signal from the body that something is wrong. Reassess the situation, communicate openly, and consider taking a break or using a smaller toy.

- **Anxiety:** Anxiety can inhibit relaxation, making fisting difficult. Incorporate relaxation techniques such as deep breathing or gentle massage to ease tension.

- **Lack of Lubrication:** Insufficient lubrication can lead to discomfort. Always keep lubricant handy and reapply as necessary.

Aftercare

Aftercare is crucial following any intense sexual experience, especially fisting. Engage in gentle aftercare practices:

- **Cuddling and Affection:** Spend time together, cuddling, and discussing the experience. This reinforces intimacy and connection.

- **Physical Care:** Check in on any physical sensations. If there's any pain or discomfort, address it with care. Consider using soothing creams or taking a warm bath.

- **Emotional Check-In:** Discuss how each partner felt during the experience. This can help process any emotions that arose and enhance future experiences.

Conclusion

Gradual and sensational fisting can be an exhilarating exploration of pleasure when approached thoughtfully. By understanding anatomy, preparing adequately, and communicating openly, partners can create a deeply intimate and fulfilling experience. Remember, the journey into fisting is as much about connection as it is about pleasure—embrace it with an open heart and mind.

Communication and Trust during Fisting

Fisting can be an exhilarating experience, but it requires a strong foundation of communication and trust between partners. This section explores the dynamics of effective communication and the importance of trust in ensuring a safe and pleasurable fisting experience.

The Importance of Communication

Communication is the cornerstone of any intimate encounter, especially when it comes to activities that may involve discomfort or risk, such as fisting. Open dialogue allows partners to express their desires, boundaries, and any concerns they may have. Here are key aspects to consider:

- **Pre-Play Discussions:** Before engaging in fisting, partners should have a candid conversation about their interests and limits. Discuss what fisting means to each partner and what they hope to experience.

- **Establishing Safe Words:** Safe words are essential in any BDSM or kink-related activity, including fisting. These words should be easy to remember and say. A common practice is to use a traffic light system: *green* for "keep going," *yellow* for "slow down," and *red* for "stop immediately."

- **Checking In:** During the act of fisting, it's important to maintain ongoing communication. Partners should check in with each other regularly to ensure comfort levels are maintained. Simple phrases like, "How are you feeling?" or "Do you want to continue?" can be very effective.

- **Post-Play Debriefing:** Aftercare is a crucial part of the fisting experience. Aftercare involves discussing what went well, what could be improved, and how each partner felt during the experience. This helps reinforce trust and emotional intimacy.

Building Trust

Trust is an essential component of any sexual activity, particularly those that involve vulnerability, such as fisting. Building trust takes time and effort, and it can be enhanced through the following practices:

- **Gradual Exploration:** Partners should start with less intense forms of anal play before progressing to fisting. This gradual approach helps build trust and allows both partners to gauge comfort levels.

- **Respecting Boundaries:** Each partner must respect the established boundaries. If one partner expresses discomfort or wants to stop, the other must honor that request without question. This respect fosters trust and safety.

- **Creating a Safe Environment:** A safe physical and emotional environment is crucial for trust. This includes ensuring the space is private, comfortable, and free from interruptions. Additionally, using safe and clean tools, such as gloves and plenty of lubricant, can enhance the feeling of safety.

- **Sharing Experiences:** Sharing past experiences related to fisting or other intimate activities can help partners understand each other's perspectives and build a stronger connection. This sharing creates empathy and reinforces trust.

Addressing Common Concerns

Even with strong communication and trust, partners may encounter challenges when engaging in fisting. Here are some common concerns and how to address them:

- **Fear of Pain or Discomfort:** One partner may fear that fisting will be painful. Openly discussing these fears can help alleviate anxiety. Partners can agree to start slowly and use plenty of lubrication to ease the process.

- **Concerns About Injury:** Fisting can carry risks if not done carefully. Partners should educate themselves about safe fisting techniques, such as using fingers that are well-lubricated and keeping nails trimmed to avoid injury.

- **Emotional Vulnerability:** Engaging in fisting can evoke strong emotions. Partners should acknowledge that feelings of vulnerability are normal and be prepared to support each other emotionally. This support can be vital in reinforcing trust.

Examples of Effective Communication

To illustrate effective communication during fisting, consider the following scenarios:

- Scenario 1: Pre-Play Communication

    Partner A: "I've been thinking about trying fisting. I'm excited but a little nervous. How do you feel about it?" Partner B: "I'm open to it! Let's talk about what we both want to explore and our limits."

- Scenario 2: In-Play Check-In

    Partner A: "I'm starting to insert my fingers now. How does that feel?" Partner B: "It feels good, but can you go a little slower?"

- Scenario 3: Post-Play Debriefing

    Partner A: "That was intense! I loved how we communicated throughout. How did you feel?" Partner B: "I felt safe and cared for. I'd love to try it again!"

Conclusion

In conclusion, effective communication and trust are paramount when engaging in fisting. By establishing clear boundaries, using safe words, and maintaining open dialogue throughout the experience, partners can create a safe and pleasurable environment. Building trust through gradual exploration, respecting boundaries, and addressing concerns will enhance the overall experience, making it more fulfilling for both partners. Remember, the key to unlocking the full potential of fisting lies in the strength of your connection and the clarity of your communication.

Exploring Power Dynamics with Anal Fisting

Anal fisting, a practice that involves the insertion of a hand into the anus, can evoke a spectrum of emotions and sensations that intertwine physical pleasure with psychological depth. This section delves into the power dynamics inherent in anal fisting, exploring how consent, trust, and communication play pivotal roles in enhancing the experience for all parties involved.

Understanding Power Dynamics

Power dynamics in sexual relationships refer to the ways in which power is negotiated and expressed between partners. In the context of anal fisting, these dynamics can manifest in various forms, including dominance and submission, trust, and vulnerability. It's essential to recognize that engaging in anal fisting can amplify feelings of surrender or control, depending on the roles assumed by participants.

Dominance and Submission The act of anal fisting can serve as a powerful expression of dominance and submission. For some, the giver may derive pleasure from the act of controlling the pace and depth of penetration, while the receiver may find joy in surrendering to that control. This interplay can be deeply satisfying, as it allows both partners to explore their desires within a framework of trust.

Establishing Trust and Consent

Before embarking on the journey of anal fisting, establishing trust and obtaining clear consent is paramount. Open communication about desires, boundaries, and limits should be prioritized. The following steps can help facilitate this process:

- **Pre-Play Discussion:** Engage in a conversation about what each partner hopes to experience. Discuss any fears or concerns, and ensure both parties feel comfortable.
- **Establishing Safe Words:** Agree on a safe word or signal that can be used if one partner feels uncomfortable or wishes to stop. This ensures that both partners can communicate their needs effectively.
- **Continuous Consent:** Consent should be ongoing. Check in with each other throughout the experience to ensure comfort levels are maintained.

Navigating Vulnerability

Engaging in anal fisting requires a significant level of vulnerability from the receiver. This vulnerability can heighten the emotional connection between partners, but it also necessitates a strong foundation of trust. The receiver must feel safe to explore their limits, knowing that their partner respects their boundaries.

Communication During Play During anal fisting, communication remains crucial. The giver should be attentive to the receiver's verbal and non-verbal cues. If the receiver expresses discomfort, it is vital to respond immediately, adjusting the approach or stopping altogether. This responsiveness reinforces trust and enhances the overall experience.

Techniques for Exploring Power Dynamics

When exploring power dynamics through anal fisting, consider the following techniques to deepen the experience:

- **Gradual Progression:** Start with gentle insertion of fingers before progressing to the fist. This gradual approach allows the receiver to acclimate to the sensation and establishes a rhythm that can be adjusted based on feedback.
- **Control and Pace:** The giver can take control of the pace, allowing the receiver to surrender to the experience. Alternating between slow, deliberate movements and more vigorous thrusts can create a dynamic interplay of power.
- **Verbal Cues:** Incorporate verbal communication as part of the experience. The giver can encourage the receiver with affirmations or instructions, enhancing the feeling of submission.

Addressing Challenges

While exploring power dynamics through anal fisting can be immensely pleasurable, it is not without challenges. Here are some common issues and strategies to address them:

Fear of Pain or Discomfort   Many individuals may feel apprehensive about the potential for pain during anal fisting. To mitigate this fear, it is essential to:

- **Prioritize Relaxation:** Engage in relaxation techniques, such as deep breathing or gentle massage, to help the receiver feel more at ease.

- **Use Plenty of Lubrication:** Adequate lubrication is critical for comfort. Opt for high-quality, body-safe lubricants to reduce friction and enhance pleasure.

- **Communicate Openly:** Encourage the receiver to voice any discomfort immediately. This open line of communication allows for adjustments to be made in real-time.

Navigating Emotional Responses   Engaging in anal fisting can evoke unexpected emotional responses, such as vulnerability, fear, or even exhilaration. It is important to:

- **Debrief After Play:** Aftercare is essential. Discuss the experience, addressing any feelings that arose during the session. This can help partners process their emotions and reinforce the bond of trust.

- **Provide Reassurance:** Offer comfort and reassurance to each other post-play. This can help mitigate any lingering feelings of vulnerability and enhance emotional intimacy.

Conclusion

Exploring power dynamics through anal fisting can be a transformative experience, merging physical pleasure with emotional depth. By prioritizing trust, communication, and consent, partners can navigate the complexities of power dynamics, enhancing both the experience and their connection. Embrace the journey, and allow yourselves to discover the profound pleasures that lie within the realms of vulnerability and surrender.

Impact Play and Anal Sex

Impact play, a thrilling exploration of sensation and power dynamics, can add an exhilarating dimension to anal sex. This section delves into the techniques, safety precautions, and psychological considerations that enhance the experience of combining impact play with anal pleasure.

Understanding Impact Play

Impact play involves striking the body in a controlled manner to create pleasurable sensations. This can include spanking, flogging, or using paddles, and is often incorporated into BDSM practices. The key to successful impact play lies in establishing trust and communication between partners, ensuring that both parties feel safe and excited about the experience.

Theoretical Framework

The pleasure derived from impact play can be understood through the lens of both physiological and psychological theories. The **Gate Control Theory** suggests that non-painful stimuli (like the sensations of impact) can inhibit the perception of pain. This means that the pleasurable sensations created through impact can coexist with the sensations of anal penetration, enhancing overall pleasure.

$$P = S - D \tag{19}$$

Where:

- P = Pleasure experienced
- S = Sensations from impact play
- D = Discomfort or pain from anal penetration

The goal is to maximize S while minimizing D, resulting in a net positive experience.

Safety Precautions

Before engaging in impact play, it is crucial to establish safety protocols. Here are some essential guidelines:

- **Communication:** Discuss desires, limits, and safe words before beginning.

- **Consent:** Ensure that all activities are consensual and agreed upon by all parties involved.

- **Safe Words:** Establish clear safe words that indicate when to slow down or stop. Common choices include "red" for stop and "yellow" for slow down.

- **Target Areas:** Aim for fleshy areas of the body, such as the buttocks, thighs, and upper back. Avoid striking areas with bones or organs, such as the spine, kidneys, or head.

- **Aftercare:** Engage in aftercare following the session to address any physical or emotional needs. This could include cuddling, talking, or applying soothing lotion to any areas that were impacted.

Techniques for Combining Impact Play and Anal Sex

When incorporating impact play into anal sex, consider the following techniques:

- **Warm-Up:** Start with gentle spanks or light slaps to warm up the body and increase blood flow. This can heighten sensitivity and prepare the body for anal play.

- **Rhythmic Play:** Establish a rhythm of impact followed by anal penetration. For example, deliver a few spanks, then insert a finger or toy, alternating between the two for varied sensations.

- **Positioning:** Experiment with different positions that allow for both anal penetration and impact play. Positions such as doggy style or bent over can facilitate this dual stimulation.

- **Toys and Implements:** Use paddles, floggers, or even your hand to create different sensations. Each tool will produce a unique feeling, enhancing the overall experience.

Challenges and Tips for Successful Integration

While combining impact play with anal sex can be incredibly pleasurable, it may also present challenges. Here are some common problems and tips for addressing them:

- **Discomfort:** If either partner experiences discomfort, pause the activity and check in. Adjust the intensity of impact or anal penetration as needed.

- **Loss of Focus:** Maintaining focus during a session can be challenging. Use deep breathing techniques to stay present and connected to your body and partner.
- **Emotional Responses:** Impact play can evoke strong emotional reactions. Be prepared to offer support and understanding during aftercare, as partners may need to process their feelings.

Examples of Impact Play and Anal Sex Scenarios

To illustrate the integration of impact play with anal sex, consider the following scenarios:

- **Spanking Before Penetration:** A partner may begin with a series of spanks to the buttocks, gradually increasing intensity. After a few minutes, they can transition to anal penetration, using the heightened sensitivity to enhance pleasure.
- **Flogging and Fingering:** While one partner is flogged, the other can insert fingers into the anus, providing a unique combination of sensations. This can lead to intense pleasure as the body responds to both stimuli.
- **Roleplay Dynamics:** Incorporate roleplay into the session, where one partner takes on a dominant role and uses impact play to assert control, followed by anal penetration to deepen the experience of submission.

Conclusion

Impact play can significantly enhance anal sex, creating a dynamic interplay of sensations that heighten pleasure and intimacy. By understanding the techniques, safety precautions, and emotional considerations involved, partners can explore this thrilling combination with confidence and joy. Remember, the key to a fulfilling experience lies in communication, consent, and mutual respect. Embrace the adventure, and let your desires guide you as you explore the exciting world of impact play and anal pleasure.

Incorporating Spanking and Impact Play into Anal Play

Spanking and impact play can be exhilarating additions to anal play, enhancing the physical sensations and emotional dynamics of the experience. This section will explore the theory behind these practices, potential challenges, and practical examples for integrating them into your anal play sessions.

Theoretical Foundations

At its core, impact play involves striking the body to elicit pleasurable sensations. When combined with anal play, the heightened anticipation and physical responses can lead to intensified pleasure. The relationship between pain and pleasure is deeply rooted in human sexuality, often described through the concept of *dual sensation*. This theory posits that the brain processes pain and pleasure through similar pathways, allowing for a unique interplay between the two.

The *Gate Control Theory* of pain suggests that the nervous system can only process a limited amount of sensory information at one time. Thus, the introduction of pleasurable sensations (from anal stimulation) can help to "gate" or reduce the perception of pain from spanking. This dynamic can create a rich tapestry of sensations that can enhance arousal and intimacy between partners.

Challenges and Considerations

While incorporating spanking and impact play can be thrilling, it is essential to approach these practices with caution. Some potential challenges include:

- **Communication:** Clear communication is vital to ensure that both partners are comfortable with the level of intensity and type of impact play being used. Establishing safe words or signals can help navigate this.

- **Physical Safety:** It is crucial to avoid striking areas that could cause injury, such as the lower back or tailbone. Focus on fleshy areas like the buttocks to minimize the risk of harm.

- **Emotional Reactions:** Impact play can evoke strong emotional responses. Partners should be prepared for potential feelings of vulnerability or discomfort and should engage in aftercare to address these feelings.

Practical Techniques

Here are some techniques for incorporating spanking and impact play into anal sessions:

1. **Warm-Up:** Begin with gentle spanks to warm up the area. This can help increase blood flow and sensitivity, preparing the body for more intense sensations.

2. **Rhythmic Spanking:** Establish a rhythm that complements the anal stimulation. For example, if one partner is using a toy or fingers for anal penetration, the other can provide rhythmic spanks to the buttocks, creating a syncopated experience that enhances arousal.

3. **Varying Intensity:** Experiment with different intensities and types of impact. Use your hand for softer spanks and switch to a paddle or flogger for more pronounced sensations. This variation can keep the experience engaging and pleasurable.

4. **Targeting Sensitivity:** Pay attention to how different areas respond to impact. The upper part of the buttocks may be more sensitive, while the lower part can handle more force. Adjust your technique based on your partner's reactions.

5. **Incorporating Breath:** Encourage your partner to focus on their breath during impact play. Deep, controlled breathing can help them manage discomfort and enhance pleasure, creating a more profound connection between the two sensations.

Examples of Impact Play Scenarios

To illustrate how to effectively incorporate spanking and impact play into anal sessions, consider the following scenarios:

- **Spanking Before Anal Play:** Start with a dedicated spanking session. Gradually increase the intensity while your partner is aroused. After a set time, transition into anal play, allowing the heightened state of arousal from the spanking to enhance the anal experience.

- **Simultaneous Stimulation:** While one partner is being penetrated anally, the other can alternate between anal stimulation and spanking. This creates a dynamic interplay of sensations that can lead to intense pleasure.

- **Role Play:** Incorporate elements of role play into your impact play. For instance, you might adopt a dominant/submissive dynamic where the dominant partner uses spanking as a form of control, enhancing the psychological aspects of the experience.

Aftercare and Reflection

Aftercare is an essential component of any intense sexual experience, particularly when incorporating impact play. Aftercare can include physical comfort, such as cuddling or applying soothing lotion to the spanked areas, as well as emotional reassurance. Engage in a debriefing session to discuss what was enjoyable, what could be improved, and how each partner felt during the experience. This practice not only fosters intimacy but also helps partners grow and learn together, enhancing future encounters.

In conclusion, incorporating spanking and impact play into anal play can create a multifaceted experience that enriches pleasure and intimacy. By understanding the theoretical foundations, addressing potential challenges, and utilizing practical techniques, partners can explore this exciting dimension of their sexual journey with confidence and creativity.

Roleplay and Power Exchange during Anal Sex

Roleplay and power exchange can add an exhilarating dimension to anal play, enhancing both the physical sensations and emotional connections between partners. This section will explore the dynamics of roleplay, the nuances of power exchange, and practical techniques to incorporate these elements safely and consensually into anal sex.

Understanding Roleplay

Roleplay involves adopting different personas or scenarios to explore fantasies and desires. In the context of anal sex, roleplay can help partners step outside their everyday identities, allowing them to engage in acts that might feel taboo or forbidden. This shift can create a heightened sense of arousal and intimacy.

Common roleplay scenarios involving anal sex include:

- **Dominant/Submissive Dynamics:** One partner takes on a dominant role, while the other embraces a submissive position. This dynamic can enhance the experience, as the dominant partner guides the submissive through the act of anal play.

- **Authority Figures:** Scenarios involving authority figures, such as a teacher and student or a boss and employee, can tap into power dynamics that heighten excitement.

- **Fantasy Characters:** Engaging in roleplay as characters from movies, books, or personal fantasies can add an imaginative layer to anal play.

Power Exchange Dynamics

Power exchange is a fundamental aspect of BDSM and can significantly enrich anal play. It involves the consensual transfer of power from one partner to another, allowing the dominant partner to take control while the submissive partner relinquishes it. This dynamic can create a deep sense of trust and intimacy.

When engaging in power exchange during anal sex, consider the following:

- **Consent and Negotiation:** Clear communication is vital. Discuss desires, limits, and safe words before engaging in any roleplay or power exchange. Establishing consent ensures that both partners feel safe and respected.

- **Trust Building:** Power exchange requires a strong foundation of trust. Engage in activities that build trust before exploring more intense anal experiences. This could include lighter forms of bondage or sensory play.

- **Aftercare:** Aftercare is essential in power exchange dynamics. Following an intense session of anal play, partners should engage in aftercare to reconnect and provide emotional support. This can include cuddling, discussing the experience, or simply being present with each other.

Practical Techniques for Roleplay and Power Exchange

To effectively incorporate roleplay and power exchange into anal sex, consider the following techniques:

1. **Setting the Scene:** Create an environment that reflects the roleplay scenario. This could involve specific costumes, props, or even lighting to enhance the atmosphere.

2. **Establishing Roles:** Clearly define the roles each partner will take on. Discuss how these roles will influence the experience, including what actions are permissible and what boundaries exist.

3. **Utilizing Safe Words:** Establish safe words or signals that either partner can use to pause or stop the action if they feel uncomfortable. Common safe words include "red" for stop and "yellow" for slow down.

4. **Incorporating Toys:** Use anal toys that align with the power dynamics at play. For example, a butt plug can symbolize submission, while a strap-on can enhance the dominant partner's role.

5. **Gradual Escalation:** Start with lighter anal play, such as external stimulation or gentle penetration, before moving to more intense actions. This gradual approach allows both partners to acclimate to the sensations and dynamics at play.

Challenges and Considerations

While roleplay and power exchange can enhance anal sex, they also come with potential challenges:

- **Miscommunication:** Lack of clear communication can lead to misunderstandings and discomfort. Regular check-ins during play can mitigate this risk.

- **Emotional Vulnerability:** Power exchange can evoke strong emotions. Be prepared for the possibility of unexpected feelings arising during or after the experience. Engage in open dialogue to address these emotions.

- **Physical Safety:** Ensure that all activities are safe and consensual. Familiarize yourself with anatomy and techniques to prevent injury during anal play.

Conclusion

Incorporating roleplay and power exchange into anal sex can lead to profoundly pleasurable experiences that deepen intimacy and trust between partners. By prioritizing consent, communication, and safety, individuals can explore their desires in a fulfilling and empowering way. Embrace the journey of exploration, and let your fantasies guide you toward new heights of pleasure.

$$P_{\text{pleasure}} = f(R, E, C) \qquad (20)$$

Where:

- P_{pleasure} = overall pleasure derived from anal play
- R = roleplay engagement level
- E = emotional connection and trust
- C = communication effectiveness

Combining Pain and Pleasure for Mind-Blowing Experiences

The intersection of pain and pleasure in sexual experiences can lead to profound sensations that transcend ordinary pleasure. This section explores the psychological and physiological aspects of combining these two elements, offering techniques, considerations, and examples to enhance your anal play.

Theoretical Foundations

The concept of combining pain and pleasure is rooted in the understanding of the body's response to stimuli. The *gate control theory of pain* posits that pain and pleasure signals can compete for attention in the nervous system. When pleasure signals are strong enough, they can effectively "close the gate" to pain signals, allowing individuals to experience heightened states of ecstasy.

$$P = f(S_p, S_d) \tag{21}$$

Where:

- P = overall pleasure experienced
- S_p = strength of pleasurable stimuli
- S_d = strength of painful stimuli

This equation suggests that the balance between pleasurable and painful stimuli can be manipulated to maximize pleasure. A careful dance between the two can lead to intense orgasms and transformative experiences.

Psychological Considerations

Before embarking on the journey of combining pain and pleasure, it is crucial to address psychological readiness. Engaging in this practice requires a strong foundation of trust, communication, and consent between partners. Here are some key psychological elements to consider:

- **Trust:** Establish a safe environment where both partners feel secure exploring their limits.
- **Communication:** Discuss desires, boundaries, and safe words to ensure both partners are on the same page.
- **Mindset:** Approach the experience with an open mind. Embrace the duality of pain and pleasure as a pathway to deeper connection.

Techniques for Combining Pain and Pleasure

1. **Impact Play:** Incorporating spanking, flogging, or paddling can introduce pleasurable pain. Start with light impacts, gradually increasing intensity as comfort levels rise. Use a safe word to ensure boundaries are respected.

2. **Temperature Play:** Experimenting with hot and cold sensations can enhance pleasure. Use ice cubes or warm oils during anal play to stimulate nerve endings and create contrasting sensations.

3. **Pressure Techniques:** Applying pressure to specific areas, such as the perineum or lower back, can create a pleasurable pain experience. Use fingers, toys, or even a partner's body to apply pressure rhythmically.

4. **Fisting:** When done with care and consent, fisting can offer a unique blend of fullness and pressure that some find pleasurable. Gradually increase the intensity and communicate throughout the process.

5. **Roleplay and Power Exchange:** Engaging in scenarios where one partner takes on a dominant role can heighten the experience of combining pain and pleasure. This dynamic allows for exploration of limits and desires in a controlled environment.

Examples of Combining Pain and Pleasure

Consider the following scenarios to illustrate the effective combination of pain and pleasure:

- Scenario 1: The Spanking Session
    - Start with gentle caresses and build anticipation.
    - Introduce light spanks, gradually increasing intensity.
    - Alternate between spanking and soothing touches to create a rhythm of pain and pleasure.

- Scenario 2: Temperature Play with Wax
    - Use body-safe candle wax to create a sensation of warmth on the skin.
    - Allow the wax to cool slightly before dripping it onto erogenous zones, including the anal area.
    - Combine this with gentle anal stimulation to amplify sensations.

- Scenario 3: Fisting with Trust

- Begin with fingers, gradually increasing the number of fingers used.
- Communicate openly about comfort levels and readiness to proceed.
- Once comfortable, slowly introduce fisting, paying attention to the partner's reactions.

Safety and Aftercare

Combining pain and pleasure requires a focus on safety to ensure a positive experience. Here are some essential safety tips:

- **Use Safe Words:** Establish clear safe words that either partner can use to pause or stop the activity if needed.
- **Check In Regularly:** Maintain open communication throughout the experience to ensure both partners are comfortable.
- **Aftercare:** After engaging in intense experiences, provide aftercare to nurture emotional and physical well-being. This can include cuddling, discussing the experience, or simply being present with one another.

Conclusion

Combining pain and pleasure in anal play can lead to transformative experiences that deepen intimacy and enhance pleasure. By understanding the theoretical foundations, employing effective techniques, and prioritizing communication and safety, you can unlock the potential for mind-blowing experiences that celebrate the duality of human sexuality. Embrace the journey, and discover the exhilarating world of pleasure that lies at the intersection of pain and ecstasy.

Techniques for Gradual and Controlled Penetration

Gradual and controlled penetration is an essential technique in anal play that emphasizes comfort, safety, and pleasure. This section will explore various methods to facilitate a smooth and enjoyable experience for all parties involved.

Understanding Gradual Penetration

Gradual penetration refers to the slow and careful introduction of objects or body parts into the anus. This technique is crucial for reducing discomfort and allowing the body to adjust to the sensations. The primary goal is to create a pleasurable experience while minimizing the risk of pain or injury.

Theoretical Framework

The anus is a sensitive area with numerous nerve endings, making it highly responsive to touch. Gradual penetration allows for the desensitization of the anal sphincter and the surrounding tissues, which can enhance pleasure over time. The following principles should guide the practice of gradual penetration:

- **Relaxation:** The receiving partner should be in a relaxed state, both physically and mentally. This can be achieved through deep breathing exercises, gentle massage, or foreplay.

- **Lubrication:** Adequate lubrication is essential to prevent friction and discomfort. Use high-quality water-based or silicone-based lubricants to ensure a smooth experience.

- **Communication:** Open and honest communication between partners is vital. Discuss desires, boundaries, and any concerns before beginning.

Techniques for Gradual Penetration

1. Finger Techniques Fingers are a versatile tool for gradual penetration. Start with one well-lubricated finger, allowing the receiving partner to control the pace.

1. **Preparation:** Ensure that both partners are comfortable and relaxed.
2. **Initial Contact:** Begin by gently massaging the external anal area to stimulate relaxation.
3. **Slow Insertion:** Gradually insert the finger, pausing frequently to allow the receiving partner to adjust.
4. **Movement:** Once fully inserted, experiment with gentle movements—circular motions or slight thrusting can enhance pleasure.

2. Use of Toys Anal toys can provide a different sensation and facilitate gradual penetration. Choose toys designed for anal use, which typically have a flared base for safety.

1. **Choosing the Right Toy:** Start with smaller toys, such as anal beads or a slim butt plug.

2. **Lubrication:** Apply a generous amount of lubricant to both the toy and the anal area.

3. **Insertion:** Begin with the smallest part of the toy, inserting it slowly while maintaining open communication.

4. **Gradual Increase:** Once the partner is comfortable, gradually increase the size of the toy or the depth of penetration.

3. **Partnered Techniques** In partnered anal play, gradual penetration can be achieved through various positions that allow for control and comfort.

1. **Spooning Position:** This position allows for intimate contact and control. The receiving partner can guide the thrusting motions, ensuring comfort.

2. **Cowgirl Position:** In this position, the receiving partner takes control, allowing them to dictate the pace and depth of penetration.

3. **Side-lying Position:** This position allows for slow penetration while providing support and comfort.

Addressing Common Problems

Despite the best intentions, challenges may arise during gradual penetration. Here are common issues and solutions:

- **Discomfort or Pain:** If discomfort occurs, stop immediately. Allow the receiving partner to take a break, and check in on their comfort level. Adjust lubrication or try a different technique.

- **Tension:** If the receiving partner feels tense, return to relaxation techniques such as breathing exercises or gentle massage.

- **Communication Breakdowns:** Establish a safe word or signal to halt penetration if discomfort arises. This promotes trust and ensures a positive experience.

Examples of Gradual Penetration Scenarios

To illustrate the techniques discussed, consider the following scenarios:

Scenario 1: Solo Play   During solo anal play, a person can use a small butt plug. They start by applying lubricant and gently inserting the toy while focusing on their breathing. They take their time, pausing frequently to allow their body to adjust.

Scenario 2: Partner Play   In a partnered scenario, one partner uses fingers to stimulate the anus. They begin with gentle external massage before gradually inserting one finger. The receiving partner communicates their comfort level, allowing for a pleasurable experience.

Conclusion

Gradual and controlled penetration is a key technique for maximizing pleasure and minimizing discomfort in anal play. By prioritizing relaxation, communication, and lubrication, partners can explore new heights of pleasure together. Remember, the journey of anal exploration should be enjoyable and consensual, fostering a deeper connection between partners.

Anal Play in BDSM

Anal Bondage Techniques

Anal bondage is a thrilling intersection of pleasure and restraint that can elevate the experience of anal play to new heights. It combines the physical sensations of bondage with the unique pleasures of anal stimulation, creating a dynamic that can enhance trust, intimacy, and exploration between partners. This section will delve into various anal bondage techniques, their theoretical underpinnings, practical considerations, and examples to inspire your journey.

Theoretical Foundations of Anal Bondage

Anal bondage operates on several psychological and physiological principles:

- **Trust and Vulnerability:** Engaging in anal bondage requires a high level of trust between partners. The submissive partner must feel safe and secure to explore their boundaries, while the dominant partner must be attuned to the needs and limits of their partner.

- **Heightened Sensation:** Restraint can amplify sensations, making anal play more intense. The inability to move freely can heighten anticipation and arousal, leading to greater pleasure.

- **Power Dynamics:** Anal bondage can incorporate elements of power exchange, where the dominant partner exerts control over the submissive partner's body. This dynamic can enhance the emotional connection and deepen the experience.

Practical Considerations

Before engaging in anal bondage, consider the following:

- **Safety:** Always prioritize safety. Use safe words and signals to ensure that both partners can communicate effectively. Establish clear boundaries and respect them at all times.
- **Equipment:** Choose appropriate bondage equipment, such as ropes, cuffs, or harnesses, that are specifically designed for safety and comfort. Avoid materials that can cause injury or discomfort.
- **Hygiene:** Maintain proper hygiene before engaging in anal bondage. Clean the anal area and any toys or equipment used to prevent infections or discomfort.

Techniques for Anal Bondage

Here are several techniques to incorporate anal bondage into your play:

1. **Basic Restraints** Using simple restraints, such as wrist or ankle cuffs, can create a sense of helplessness that enhances anal stimulation. Position the submissive partner in a way that allows for easy access to the anal area while ensuring comfort.

- **Example:** Have the submissive partner lie on their back with their wrists bound above their head. This position allows for easy access to the anal area while also exposing the body for additional stimulation.

2. **Rope Bondage** Rope bondage offers versatility and creativity. Use soft, flexible ropes to create intricate patterns that not only restrain but also stimulate the skin.

- **Example:** The "Hogtie" position can be particularly effective. Bind the wrists and ankles together behind the back, creating a sense of vulnerability. This position allows for easy access to both the anal area and other erogenous zones.

3. Spreader Bars   Spreader bars can be used to hold the legs apart, providing unobstructed access to the anal area. This technique can enhance the feeling of exposure and vulnerability.

- **Example:** Attach the spreader bar to the ankles of the submissive partner while they lie on their stomach. This position allows for easy access for anal play while also creating a visually stimulating scene.

4. Anal Plug Bondage   Incorporating anal plugs into bondage can enhance the experience. The feeling of fullness combined with restraint can lead to heightened pleasure.

- **Example:** Insert a comfortable anal plug before binding the partner. The combination of the plug and restraints can create a powerful sense of pleasure and anticipation.

5. Sensation Play   Combine anal bondage with sensation play, using feathers, ice, or other sensory tools to heighten arousal. The contrast of sensations can create an exhilarating experience.

- **Example:** While the submissive partner is restrained, use a feather or ice cube to tease the skin around the anal area, building anticipation before engaging in anal play.

Common Problems and Solutions

1. Discomfort or Pain   If either partner experiences discomfort during anal bondage, it is essential to stop immediately.

- **Solution:** Discuss any discomfort openly and adjust the restraints or positions as necessary. Ensure that both partners are comfortable and enjoying the experience.

2. Communication Breakdowns   Effective communication is vital in anal bondage. Misunderstandings can lead to discomfort or unsafe situations.

- **Solution:** Establish clear safe words and signals before beginning. Regularly check in with each other to ensure both partners are comfortable and enjoying the experience.

3. **Equipment Issues**   Using inappropriate or unsafe equipment can lead to injury.

- ✦ **Solution:** Always use equipment designed for bondage and anal play. Check for any wear and tear before use, and ensure that all materials are safe for the body.

Conclusion

Anal bondage techniques can provide an exciting and pleasurable dimension to anal play. By understanding the theoretical foundations, prioritizing safety, and exploring various techniques, partners can create a rich and fulfilling experience. Remember, the key to successful anal bondage lies in trust, communication, and a shared desire to explore the boundaries of pleasure together. Embrace the adventure, and let your fantasies unfold.

Introduction to Anal Bondage

Anal bondage is a thrilling and intimate practice that combines the excitement of restraint with the unique sensations of anal play. It is an intersection of two powerful elements: the physical and psychological aspects of bondage and the heightened sensations associated with anal stimulation. This section will explore the principles of anal bondage, address common challenges, and provide practical examples to enhance your experience.

The Philosophy of Anal Bondage

At its core, anal bondage is about trust, consent, and exploration. It allows partners to explore their boundaries and desires in a safe and controlled environment. The philosophy behind anal bondage is rooted in the understanding that pleasure can be derived from both the act of restraint and the sensations that come from anal stimulation.

Bondage can create a sense of vulnerability and surrender, which can heighten arousal. When one partner is restrained, they often feel more open to experiencing new sensations, while the partner in control can derive pleasure from both the act of bondage and the pleasure they give.

Safety Considerations

Before engaging in anal bondage, it is crucial to prioritize safety. Here are some key considerations:

- **Consent:** Always ensure that both partners are fully consenting to the experience. Discuss limits, desires, and safe words prior to engaging in anal bondage.

- **Safety Equipment:** Use appropriate bondage gear, such as soft restraints or specialized anal bondage equipment. Avoid using items that can cause injury or discomfort.

- **Monitoring:** Keep an eye on your partner's physical and emotional state throughout the experience. If they show signs of distress, be prepared to stop immediately.

- **Hygiene:** Ensure that all equipment is clean and safe for use, particularly when involving anal play. Consider using gloves and ensuring that anal toys are sanitized.

Common Challenges

While anal bondage can be exhilarating, it can also present challenges. Here are some common issues that practitioners may face:

- **Fear of Pain:** Many individuals fear that anal bondage will lead to discomfort or pain. Open communication about fears and desires can help alleviate these concerns.

- **Physical Discomfort:** Restraint can sometimes lead to physical discomfort. It is essential to choose the right bondage techniques and equipment to ensure comfort.

- **Emotional Vulnerability:** Engaging in anal bondage can evoke strong emotions. It is important to establish a safe word and debrief after the experience to address any feelings that may arise.

Examples of Anal Bondage Techniques

Here are some practical examples of anal bondage techniques that can enhance pleasure and connection:

Basic Restraint Start with simple restraints, such as wrist or ankle cuffs. Secure your partner in a comfortable position that allows for easy access to the anal area. This can enhance feelings of vulnerability and excitement.

Positioning Experiment with different positions that facilitate anal play while incorporating bondage. For example, the "doggy style" position can be enhanced by restraining the wrists or ankles, allowing for deeper penetration and heightened sensations.

Sensory Deprivation Incorporate blindfolds or earplugs to heighten the experience. By limiting your partner's senses, they may become more attuned to the sensations of anal play, making the experience more intense.

Use of Toys Integrate anal toys into your bondage play. For instance, using a butt plug while your partner is restrained can create an exciting combination of sensations. Ensure that the toy is securely in place and that you can easily remove it if necessary.

Role Play Incorporate elements of role play into your anal bondage experience. By establishing a power dynamic, you can explore fantasies that enhance the pleasure derived from both bondage and anal stimulation.

Conclusion

Anal bondage is an empowering practice that can deepen intimacy and enhance pleasure. By understanding the principles of safety, communication, and consent, you can explore this thrilling aspect of sexual expression. Embrace the journey of discovery and enjoy the unique sensations that anal bondage can offer.

Equipment and Safety Precautions

When delving into the world of anal play, especially within the context of BDSM, understanding the necessary equipment and adhering to safety precautions is paramount. This section will provide an overview of the essential tools, their uses, and the best practices to ensure a pleasurable and safe experience.

Essential Equipment for Anal Play

Engaging in anal play, particularly in a BDSM context, requires specific equipment designed to enhance pleasure while prioritizing safety. Here are some key items to consider:

- **Lubricants:** Anal play necessitates ample lubrication due to the lack of natural moisture in the anal area. Silicone-based lubricants are often recommended for their long-lasting properties, while water-based lubricants are easier to clean but may require reapplication. Avoid oil-based lubricants with latex condoms, as they can cause breakage.

- **Anal Toys:** There is a wide variety of anal toys available, including anal beads, butt plugs, and prostate massagers. When selecting toys, ensure they have a flared base to prevent them from becoming lost inside the body. Materials such as silicone, glass, and stainless steel are preferred for their body-safe properties.

- **Fisting Gloves:** For those exploring fisting, using gloves can enhance safety and hygiene. Latex or nitrile gloves provide a barrier that can prevent the transmission of bacteria and make cleanup easier.

- **Restraints and Bondage Gear:** If incorporating anal play into BDSM, restraints such as cuffs, ropes, or bondage tape can be used to enhance the experience. Ensure that any restraints used are designed for safety and comfort, allowing for easy release if necessary.

- **Impact Toys:** If including impact play, items like paddles, floggers, or crops can be used. Ensure that the materials are safe for use on the body and that the intensity of impact is consensually agreed upon.

Safety Precautions

Safety is of utmost importance in any sexual practice, but it becomes even more critical when engaging in anal play, especially in a BDSM context. Here are essential safety precautions to consider:

- **Communication:** Prior to any anal play, it is crucial to have an open and honest discussion with your partner(s) about desires, limits, and boundaries. Establish safe words or signals to ensure that everyone can communicate effectively during the experience.

- **Hygiene:** Maintaining cleanliness is vital to prevent infections. Before engaging in anal play, both partners should wash their hands and any toys used. If using fingers, ensure that nails are trimmed and smooth to avoid injury.

- **Gradual Exploration:** Start slowly when engaging in anal play. Begin with external stimulation and gradually work towards insertion. This approach allows the body to adjust and reduces the risk of discomfort or injury.

- **Use of Safe Words:** Establishing safe words is essential, especially in BDSM contexts. A safe word should be easy to remember and say, allowing for immediate communication if anyone feels uncomfortable or needs to stop.

- **Understanding Anatomy:** Familiarize yourself with the anatomy of the anal region. Knowing the location of sensitive areas and understanding how to stimulate them can enhance pleasure while minimizing the risk of injury.

- **Avoiding Alcohol and Drugs:** While some may feel that substances enhance pleasure, they can impair judgment and communication. It is best to engage in anal play when both partners are sober and able to communicate clearly.

- **Aftercare:** Aftercare is an essential part of any BDSM experience. Following anal play, take time to check in with your partner, provide comfort, and discuss the experience. This helps reinforce trust and connection.

- **Emergency Preparedness:** Be aware of potential risks associated with anal play, including tearing or bleeding. Have a first aid kit on hand, and know how to respond to common injuries. If significant pain or bleeding occurs, seek medical attention.

Conclusion

By understanding the necessary equipment and implementing safety precautions, individuals can explore anal play with confidence and care. Embracing these practices not only enhances the experience but also fosters a deeper connection between partners. Remember, the key to pleasurable anal play lies in communication, consent, and respect for each other's boundaries.

Techniques for Anal Bondage and Control

Anal bondage is an exhilarating practice that combines the thrill of restraint with the unique sensations of anal play. It requires a deep understanding of both the physical and psychological aspects of bondage, as well as a commitment to safety and consent. This section will explore various techniques for anal bondage and control, focusing on practical applications, safety considerations, and the dynamics of power exchange.

Understanding Anal Bondage

Anal bondage involves the use of restraints to limit movement, enhancing the sensations experienced during anal play. The psychological aspect of bondage can heighten arousal, as surrendering control can lead to deeper trust and intimacy between partners. Key principles of anal bondage include:

- **Consent:** Always ensure that all parties involved have given informed consent. Discuss limits, safe words, and aftercare before engaging in any bondage activities.

- **Safety:** Use safe materials for restraints (e.g., soft ropes, cuffs) and avoid putting pressure on sensitive areas. Regularly check in with your partner to ensure their comfort and safety.

- **Communication:** Maintain open lines of communication throughout the experience. Non-verbal cues may also be necessary, especially when the partner is restrained.

Basic Techniques for Anal Bondage

1. Using Ropes Rope bondage can be an effective way to restrain a partner while allowing for versatility in positioning. Start with basic knots that can be easily undone in case of emergency. A popular technique is the *Hogtie*, which binds the wrists and ankles together.

Hogtie: Secure wrists and ankles with rope, ensuring comfort and mobility.
(22)

This position can enhance the sensations of anal play, as the partner is fully restrained and vulnerable.

2. Cuffs and Harnesses Using cuffs or harnesses designed for bondage can provide a more secure and comfortable experience. These devices can be adjusted for snugness without restricting circulation.

Cuffs: Soft cuffs can be placed on wrists and ankles, allowing for movement while mainta
(23)

A popular harness for anal bondage is the *Chest Harness*, which can keep a partner upright while allowing for easy access to their body.

3. **Positioning for Control**   The position in which a partner is restrained can significantly affect the experience of anal play. Consider the following positions:

- **Face Down:** This position allows for easy access to the anus while keeping the partner's body exposed. It can be achieved by binding the wrists behind the back and securing the ankles.
- **Kneeling:** Binding the partner's hands above their head while they kneel creates an open posture for anal play. This position can enhance feelings of submission.
- **Over the Edge:** Have the partner bend over a bed or table, securing their wrists and ankles. This position offers deep access and control.

Advanced Techniques for Sensation and Control

1. Anal Hooking   Anal hooking is an advanced technique that involves the use of specialized hooks designed for anal play. These hooks can provide a unique sensation and can be used to control the partner's movements.

Anal Hook: Insert a hook designed for anal play, securing it to a point of restraint.

(24)

Ensure that the hook is made from body-safe materials and is used with caution.

2. Temperature Play   Incorporating temperature play into anal bondage can heighten sensations. Use warm or cool objects (e.g., glass toys, heated elements) during bondage to stimulate the area.

Temperature Play: Apply warm or cool objects to the anal area while restrained.

(25)

This can increase arousal and create a more intense experience.

3. Sensation Control   Using blindfolds or sensory deprivation can enhance the experience of anal bondage. By removing sight, partners may become more attuned to touch, sound, and other sensations.

Sensation Control: Blindfold the partner to enhance their experience of anal stimulation.

(26)

Safety Considerations

When engaging in anal bondage, it is crucial to prioritize safety. Here are some essential safety tips:

- **Check for Circulation:** Regularly check that restraints are not cutting off circulation. Look for signs of discoloration or numbness.

- **Have Safety Scissors Ready:** Always have a pair of safety scissors on hand to quickly cut restraints if necessary.

- **Establish Safe Words:** Create clear safe words that can be used to pause or stop the activity immediately.

Conclusion

Anal bondage can be a thrilling addition to your sexual repertoire, enhancing both pleasure and intimacy. By understanding the techniques, safety considerations, and dynamics of power exchange, you can create a fulfilling and empowering experience for both you and your partner. Remember, the key to successful anal bondage lies in consent, communication, and care. Embrace the journey of exploration and enjoy the depths of pleasure that anal bondage can offer.

Anal Torture and Sensation Play

Anal torture and sensation play is a thrilling exploration of the boundaries of pleasure and pain, allowing individuals to engage in experiences that heighten sensitivity, arousal, and intimacy. This section delves into the theory behind sensation play, the challenges it may present, and practical examples to enhance your understanding and enjoyment of this daring practice.

Understanding Anal Torture and Sensation Play

Sensation play involves the use of various techniques to stimulate the body's nerve endings, creating intense feelings that can range from pleasurable to painful. Anal torture, in this context, refers specifically to the application of these techniques to the anal area, often pushing the limits of comfort and pleasure. The psychological and physiological aspects of sensation play are crucial to its enjoyment and safety.

Theoretical Framework The foundation of sensation play lies in the concept of *sensory overload*, where the nervous system is bombarded with stimuli that can lead to heightened arousal. This is often accompanied by the release of endorphins, which can create a euphoric state, sometimes referred to as a *subspace*.

The following equation illustrates the relationship between arousal and sensation:

$$A = f(S, P, E) \tag{27}$$

Where:

- A = Arousal level
- S = Sensation intensity
- P = Psychological state (trust, safety)
- E = Environmental factors (setting, mood)

This equation emphasizes that arousal is a function of both physical sensations and psychological factors, highlighting the importance of consent and communication in any anal torture scenario.

Common Techniques for Anal Torture

1. **Temperature Play**: Utilizing heat and cold to stimulate the anal area can create contrasting sensations that enhance arousal. Ice cubes or heated toys can be used for this purpose. Always ensure that the temperature is safe to avoid burns or frostbite.

2. **Pressure and Weight**: Applying pressure to the anal area using various objects (e.g., weighted toys or hands) can intensify sensations. Experiment with different weights and pressures to find what feels best.

3. **Electro-Stimulation**: Devices designed for electrostimulation can provide a unique blend of pleasure and pain. These devices send small electrical currents through the anal area, stimulating nerve endings in unexpected ways. Always start with low settings and gradually increase intensity.

4. **Vibrators and Probes**: Using vibrating anal toys can create a range of sensations. The vibrations can be adjusted to different frequencies and intensities, allowing for tailored experiences.

5. **Impact Play**: Incorporating light spanking or the use of paddles can heighten sensations in the anal area. The key is to maintain open communication with your partner about their comfort levels and boundaries.

Challenges and Safety Precautions

While anal torture and sensation play can be exhilarating, it is essential to approach these practices with caution:

- **Communication**: Always discuss desires, limits, and safe words before engaging in anal torture. Establishing a clear line of communication ensures that both partners feel safe and respected.
- **Consent**: Consent must be enthusiastic and ongoing. Both partners should feel empowered to stop or adjust the intensity of play at any time.
- **Hygiene**: Maintaining cleanliness is crucial when engaging in anal play. Ensure that all toys and body parts are clean before and after play to prevent infections.
- **Physical Limitations**: Be aware of your and your partner's physical limits. Pain thresholds can vary significantly between individuals, so start slowly and gauge reactions.
- **Aftercare**: Aftercare is vital in sensation play. Providing emotional and physical support after an intense session helps partners reconnect and process the experience.

Examples of Anal Torture Scenarios

1. **The Temperature Experiment**: Begin with a heated anal plug, allowing the warmth to spread. Follow this with an ice cube gently applied to the area, alternating between hot and cold to create a thrilling contrast.
2. **Weighted Exploration**: Use a series of progressively heavier anal toys. Start with a light toy and gradually increase the weight, allowing your partner to express their comfort levels throughout the process.
3. **Electric Excitement**: Introduce an electro-stimulation device with adjustable settings. Start at the lowest level, allowing your partner to acclimate before experimenting with higher settings.
4. **Impact Play Dynamics**: Incorporate a light spanking session, alternating between gentle taps and firmer strikes. Communicate throughout to ensure the experience remains pleasurable and consensual.

Conclusion

Anal torture and sensation play can be a deeply rewarding experience when approached with care, consent, and creativity. By understanding the theoretical underpinnings, employing various techniques, and maintaining open communication, you can unlock new dimensions of pleasure and intimacy.

Embrace the exploration of your desires, and remember that the journey is as important as the destination.

Understanding Different Types of Sensation Play

Sensation play encompasses a wide range of activities designed to heighten the physical and emotional experiences of those involved. It invites participants to explore the boundaries of pleasure and discomfort, utilizing various stimuli to achieve heightened arousal and intimacy. This section delves into the different types of sensation play, their theoretical underpinnings, potential challenges, and practical examples.

Theoretical Framework

At its core, sensation play is rooted in the principles of BDSM (Bondage, Discipline, Dominance, Submission, Sadism, and Masochism). It operates on the premise that pleasure and pain are not mutually exclusive; rather, they can coexist and enhance one another. The theory of **dual sensation** suggests that the body's response to pain can trigger the release of endorphins, leading to a pleasurable high. This phenomenon is often referred to as the **endorphin rush**, which can amplify the overall experience of intimacy and connection between partners.

The **gate control theory of pain** also plays a crucial role in understanding sensation play. This theory posits that the perception of pain can be modulated by the brain's processing of sensory information. When engaging in sensation play, the introduction of pleasurable stimuli can effectively "close the gate" to pain sensations, allowing individuals to experience a more profound sense of pleasure.

Types of Sensation Play

There are several types of sensation play, each offering unique experiences and opportunities for exploration. Below are some of the most common forms:

- **Temperature Play:** This involves the use of hot or cold objects to create contrasting sensations on the skin. Ice cubes, warm wax, or heated massage stones can be used to heighten sensitivity and arousal. For example, running an ice cube along the spine can create a thrilling contrast when followed by the warmth of a partner's hands.

- **Impact Play:** This includes activities such as spanking, flogging, or whipping, where the focus is on delivering controlled strikes to the body. The sensation of impact can range from a light tap to a more intense strike, allowing for a spectrum of experiences. Effective communication is crucial to ensure that both partners are comfortable with the intensity of the impact.

+ **Pressure Play:** This type of sensation play involves applying varying degrees of pressure to different parts of the body. Techniques can include squeezing, pinching, or even using tools like clamps or weights. The goal is to explore how different pressures can elicit different sensations, ranging from pleasurable to intense.

+ **Sensory Deprivation:** By limiting one or more senses, such as sight or hearing, participants can heighten their remaining senses. Blindfolds, earplugs, or hoods can be used to create an environment of sensory deprivation. This can lead to increased sensitivity to touch and heightened anticipation, intensifying the overall experience.

+ **Tickling:** This playful form of sensation play can elicit laughter and joy, while also creating a sense of vulnerability. Tickling can be a form of teasing and can be combined with other types of sensation play for a more layered experience.

+ **Role Play and Psychological Play:** Incorporating elements of fantasy and power dynamics can enhance sensation play. Engaging in role play allows partners to explore different personas and scenarios, which can heighten emotional and physical sensations. The psychological aspect of sensation play can be just as powerful as the physical sensations themselves.

Challenges and Considerations

While sensation play can be a thrilling and enriching experience, it is essential to be aware of potential challenges:

+ **Communication:** Open and honest communication is vital for ensuring that both partners feel safe and comfortable. Discussing boundaries, limits, and safe words beforehand can help prevent misunderstandings and enhance trust.

+ **Consent:** All forms of sensation play must be consensual. Consent should be enthusiastic, informed, and can be revoked at any time. Establishing a clear framework for consent before engaging in sensation play is crucial.

- **Physical Safety:** Some forms of sensation play, particularly impact play or temperature play, carry risks of injury if not executed correctly. It is essential to educate oneself on safe practices, including proper techniques and equipment usage.

- **Emotional Aftercare:** After engaging in intense sensation play, partners may experience a range of emotions. Providing aftercare—comforting, nurturing, and discussing the experience—can help partners process their feelings and reinforce the emotional connection.

Practical Examples

To illustrate the various types of sensation play, consider the following examples:

- **Temperature Play Example:** Fill a bowl with ice cubes and allow your partner to hold one while you gently run your fingers along their skin. Alternate between the cold ice and your warm hands to create a thrilling contrast that heightens sensitivity.

- **Impact Play Example:** Use a soft flogger to deliver gentle strikes across your partner's back. Start slowly, gauging their reactions, and gradually increase the intensity as they become more comfortable and responsive.

- **Sensory Deprivation Example:** Blindfold your partner and guide them through a series of sensations, such as feather-light touches, gentle pinches, or the sound of a soft whisper. The lack of sight can amplify their awareness of touch and sound, leading to heightened arousal.

- **Tickling Example:** Engage in playful tickling, focusing on sensitive areas such as the sides or underarms. Use laughter as a way to connect and build intimacy, while also exploring the boundaries of vulnerability.

Conclusion

Understanding different types of sensation play opens the door to a world of exploration and intimacy. By engaging with the body's responses to various stimuli, partners can deepen their connection and enhance their sexual experiences. As with all forms of sexual exploration, the key to successful sensation play lies in communication, consent, and a mutual understanding of boundaries. Embrace the journey of sensation play, and allow it to transform your intimate encounters into unforgettable experiences.

Techniques for Intense Anal Sensation Play

Anal sensation play is an exhilarating journey into the depths of pleasure that goes beyond mere penetration. It involves stimulating the sensitive nerve endings around the anus and within the anal cavity to create a range of sensations, from gentle teasing to intense pleasure. This section will explore various techniques and methods that can heighten the experience of anal sensation play.

Understanding Sensation Play

Sensation play in the anal region can be categorized into two main types: **direct stimulation** and **indirect stimulation**. Direct stimulation involves applying pressure or movement to the anal area itself, while indirect stimulation may include teasing surrounding areas or using temperature and texture to enhance the overall experience.

1. Temperature Play

One of the most effective ways to enhance anal sensation is through temperature play. This can involve using hot or cold objects to stimulate the skin and heighten sensitivity.

- **Cold Play:** Ice cubes or chilled metal toys can be used to create a shocking contrast against warm skin. The sudden cold can evoke strong sensations and enhance arousal. Be sure to wrap ice cubes in a soft cloth to prevent direct contact with the skin, which can lead to discomfort or injury.

- **Warm Play:** Warm towels or heated toys can provide a soothing sensation, relaxing the muscles and enhancing pleasure. Always test the temperature on your wrist before applying it to sensitive areas.

2. Texture Play

Using objects with varying textures can stimulate the anal area in unique ways. The key is to explore different materials that can provide contrasting sensations:

- **Rough Textures:** Items like textured anal beads or ribbed toys can create a stimulating feeling as they move in and out. The added friction can enhance pleasure during penetration.

- **Smooth Textures:** Smooth toys or fingers can provide a different experience, allowing for gentle gliding motions that can be both soothing and pleasurable. Experiment with different speeds and pressures to find what feels best.

3. Vibration Play

Incorporating vibrational elements can significantly enhance anal sensation. Many anal toys come with built-in vibrators, but you can also use external devices:

- **Vibrating Toys:** Choose toys specifically designed for anal use that have varying vibration patterns. Start with lower settings and gradually increase intensity as comfort allows.
- **External Vibrators:** Placing a small, external vibrator against the perineum can stimulate both the anal and genital areas simultaneously, creating a more intense experience.

4. Pressure Play

Applying varying degrees of pressure can lead to profound sensations. This can be done through:

- **Fingers:** Use your fingers to apply pressure around the anal opening, gradually pushing inward. Experiment with different angles and speeds to discover what elicits the most pleasure.
- **Toys:** Use toys designed for anal play that allow for controlled pressure. Slowly insert and remove the toy while varying the angle and depth of penetration.

5. Mindful Breathing and Relaxation Techniques

Before engaging in intense anal sensation play, it is crucial to relax the body and mind. This can be achieved through:

- **Deep Breathing:** Encourage relaxation by taking deep, slow breaths. Inhale deeply through the nose, hold for a moment, and exhale slowly through the mouth. This can help ease tension in the body.
- **Progressive Muscle Relaxation:** Focus on tensing and then relaxing different muscle groups in the body, starting from the toes and working your way up to the head. This can help release any built-up tension.

6. Incorporating Role Play and Fantasy

Integrating role play and fantasy elements can heighten arousal and create a more immersive experience. Consider:

- **Setting the Scene:** Create an environment that enhances the mood. Dim lighting, soft music, and the right props can set the stage for intense sensation play.

- **Role Play Scenarios:** Engaging in fantasies can amplify excitement. Discuss and explore various scenarios that both partners find appealing, ensuring that communication remains open and consensual.

7. Communication and Feedback

Finally, effective communication is key to successful anal sensation play. Establish safe words and signals to ensure that both partners feel comfortable and can express their limits. Regularly check in with each other to gauge comfort levels and adjust techniques accordingly.

$$\text{Pleasure} = f(\text{Communication, Trust, Exploration}) \tag{28}$$

Where:

- f represents the function that captures the relationship between the variables.

- Pleasure increases with higher levels of Communication, Trust, and Exploration.

Conclusion

Techniques for intense anal sensation play are as diverse as the individuals who engage in them. By exploring temperature, texture, vibration, pressure, and incorporating mindfulness and communication, partners can unlock a world of pleasure that transcends conventional boundaries. Remember, the journey into anal sensation is personal and should always prioritize consent, safety, and mutual enjoyment. Embrace the adventure, and let your desires guide you into new realms of pleasure.

Combining Sensation Play with Roleplay and Power Exchange

Sensation play, roleplay, and power exchange are three integral components of BDSM that can enhance the experience of anal play. When combined thoughtfully, they can create a rich tapestry of pleasure, trust, and exploration. This section delves into the theoretical underpinnings of these practices, potential challenges, and practical examples to guide you in integrating these elements into your anal play sessions.

Theoretical Framework

At the core of combining sensation play with roleplay and power exchange lies the concept of **consensual dynamics.** This involves an agreement between participants to explore power imbalances in a safe and consensual manner. The *Dominant* (Dom) and *Submissive* (Sub) roles can significantly influence the emotional and psychological landscape of the experience, enhancing the physical sensations involved in anal play.

The **theory of arousal** suggests that heightened emotional states can amplify physical sensations. As such, engaging in roleplay—whether it be fantasy scenarios, character play, or power dynamics—can elevate the intensity of sensations experienced during anal play. This is often linked to the *psychological arousal* associated with the roles being enacted, which can lead to increased pleasure and satisfaction.

Challenges and Considerations

While the combination of these elements can be exhilarating, it is not without its challenges. Here are some potential problems to consider:

- **Miscommunication:** Clear communication is paramount in any BDSM scenario. Misunderstandings about roles, limits, or desires can lead to discomfort or harm.

- **Emotional Triggers:** Roleplay scenarios can sometimes evoke past traumas or emotional responses. It is crucial to have a thorough understanding of each participant's boundaries and triggers.

- **Safety Concerns:** Sensation play often involves the use of implements that can cause pain or discomfort. It is essential to incorporate safety measures and safe words to ensure that all parties feel secure.

Practical Examples

To effectively combine sensation play with roleplay and power exchange, consider the following examples:

Example 1: The Sensual Teacher and Eager Student In this scenario, one partner takes on the role of a strict teacher while the other embodies a willing student. The Dom might use a variety of sensation play techniques, such as gentle spanking or temperature play with ice and heat, to heighten the experience. The key here is to maintain the power dynamic, with the teacher guiding the student through their journey of pleasure. Safe words should be established, allowing the student to express their comfort level throughout the session.

Example 2: The Captive and the Captor This roleplay scenario involves a clear power exchange, with one partner acting as the captor and the other as the captive. Sensation play can be introduced through bondage techniques, such as tying the captive's hands or using blindfolds to heighten anticipation. The captor can then explore anal play with fingers or toys, combining the thrill of submission with the physical sensations of anal pleasure. Establishing limits and aftercare protocols is vital to ensure emotional safety.

Example 3: The Doctor and Patient In a medical roleplay scenario, one partner assumes the role of a doctor, while the other plays the patient. The doctor can use various tools for sensation play, such as temperature probes or anal toys, to create a clinical yet intimate atmosphere. This scenario allows for exploration of vulnerability and trust, as the patient submits to the doctor's examination. Consent and communication remain paramount, with both partners agreeing on the boundaries of the roleplay.

Conclusion

Combining sensation play with roleplay and power exchange can lead to profound experiences of pleasure, intimacy, and exploration. By understanding the theoretical aspects, addressing potential challenges, and employing practical examples, you can create enriching and memorable anal play sessions. Remember that the foundation of these practices lies in consent, communication, and mutual respect. Embrace the journey, and allow your fantasies to unfold within the safe space you create together.

Anal Training and Slavery

Anal training is a consensual practice that involves gradually increasing the size and intensity of anal play to enhance pleasure and comfort over time. It is often integrated into the dynamics of BDSM, where power exchange plays a significant role. This section explores the art of anal training, the psychological and physical aspects involved, and the responsibilities of both the trainer and the trainee in a consensual slavery context.

The Art of Anal Training

Anal training is not merely about physical preparation; it is a journey that encompasses trust, communication, and mutual respect. The primary goal is to allow the trainee to experience increased pleasure through expanded anal capacity while maintaining a focus on safety and consent.

Gradual Progression The key to successful anal training lies in gradual progression. This involves starting with smaller toys or fingers and slowly increasing the size as comfort and experience grow. A common practice is to follow the "two-week rule," where the trainee uses a specific size for two weeks before moving on to a larger option. This timeline allows the body to adapt and reduces the risk of injury.

$$\text{Size}_{\text{next}} = \text{Size}_{\text{current}} + \Delta \tag{29}$$

where Δ represents a small increment in size that the trainee feels comfortable with.

Communication and Consent Effective communication is vital in anal training. Both partners must openly discuss desires, limits, and boundaries. Establishing a safe word is crucial, allowing the trainee to signal if they feel uncomfortable or need to stop.

Building Slave Skills through Consensual Anal Play

In the context of BDSM, anal training can be intertwined with the dynamics of slavery. The trainer (dominant) assumes a guiding role, while the trainee (submissive) willingly submits to the process. This dynamic can enhance the experience, creating a deeper emotional and psychological connection.

Establishing Protocols For anal training to be effective, establishing clear protocols is essential. This includes:

- **Frequency of Training Sessions:** Determine how often training will occur (e.g., daily, weekly).
- **Types of Toys:** Agree on which toys will be used, starting from smaller sizes to larger ones.
- **Post-Session Care:** Discuss aftercare practices to ensure the trainee feels safe and cared for after each session.

Trust and Vulnerability The act of anal training can evoke feelings of vulnerability. The trainee must trust their partner to guide them through the process safely. This trust is built through consistent communication, respect for boundaries, and aftercare practices that reinforce the emotional bond.

Establishing Protocols and Punishments

In a consensual slavery dynamic, anal training may also involve protocols and punishments. These elements must be negotiated and agreed upon beforehand to ensure they enhance the experience rather than cause harm or discomfort.

Protocols Protocols can include specific behaviors that the submissive must adhere to during training sessions. For example:

- **Preparation Rituals:** The submissive may have a specific routine they follow to prepare for anal training, enhancing the psychological aspect of submission.
- **Reporting:** After each session, the submissive may be required to report their feelings, physical sensations, and any challenges they faced.

Punishments Punishments should be consensual and agreed upon in advance. They can serve as a motivational tool for the submissive to adhere to the training protocols. Examples may include:

- **Extended Training Sessions:** If the submissive does not meet the agreed-upon goals, the trainer may extend the duration of the next session.
- **Additional Tasks:** Assigning extra tasks or chores as a form of discipline can reinforce the power dynamic.

Safety Considerations

Safety is paramount in anal training and slavery. Both partners must prioritize physical and emotional well-being throughout the process.

Physical Safety

- **Hygiene:** Ensure cleanliness before and after anal play to prevent infections.
- **Lubrication:** Use plenty of high-quality lubricant to facilitate comfortable penetration and reduce the risk of injury.
- **Listening to the Body:** The submissive should always listen to their body and communicate any discomfort immediately.

Emotional Safety

- **Aftercare:** Aftercare is crucial for emotional safety. It may include cuddling, discussing the session, or engaging in comforting activities.
- **Debriefing:** After each training session, both partners should engage in a debriefing conversation to discuss what worked, what didn't, and how to improve the experience.

Conclusion

Anal training within a slavery context can be a deeply rewarding experience that enhances pleasure, intimacy, and trust between partners. By focusing on gradual progression, establishing clear protocols, and prioritizing safety and communication, both the trainer and the trainee can embark on a fulfilling journey of exploration and empowerment. Embracing the roles of trainer and trainee can lead to profound personal growth and a deeper understanding of desires, limits, and the beauty of consensual anal play.

The Art of Anal Training

Anal training is a process that involves gradually increasing the size and intensity of anal play to enhance pleasure and comfort. It requires patience, communication, and a deep understanding of one's body. This section will explore the theory behind anal training, common challenges faced, and practical examples to help individuals and couples embark on this exciting journey.

Understanding Anal Training

Anal training is based on the principle of gradual adaptation. The anal sphincter, composed of internal and external muscles, can be trained to accommodate larger objects over time. This is akin to weight training, where muscles are progressively challenged to increase strength and endurance. The goal of anal training is to enhance pleasure, comfort, and control during anal play.

Theoretical Framework

The theory behind anal training can be understood through the following key concepts:

- **Progressive Overload:** Just as muscles grow stronger with increased resistance, the anal sphincter can be conditioned to accept larger sizes through gradual exposure.

- **Neuroplasticity:** The brain's ability to adapt and reorganize itself is crucial in anal training. Positive experiences can reshape one's perception of anal play, turning initial discomfort into pleasure.

- **Mind-Body Connection:** Understanding the psychological aspects of anal training is essential. Trust, relaxation, and communication with a partner can significantly impact the training process.

Common Challenges

While anal training can be a rewarding experience, it is not without challenges. Some common issues include:

- **Pain and Discomfort:** Initial attempts at anal play may lead to pain if the body is not adequately prepared. It is crucial to listen to your body and proceed at a comfortable pace.

- **Psychological Barriers:** Fear, anxiety, and societal stigma can hinder the anal training process. Addressing these feelings through open communication and education is vital.

- **Physical Limitations:** Each individual's anatomy is different. Some may find it more challenging to accommodate larger objects due to anatomical differences. Understanding one's body is essential.

Practical Steps for Anal Training

The following steps outline a practical approach to anal training:

1. **Start Small:** Begin with smaller anal toys or fingers. The goal is to become accustomed to the sensation of fullness without discomfort.

2. **Use Plenty of Lubrication:** Adequate lubrication is crucial for comfort and safety. Water-based or silicone-based lubricants are recommended to reduce friction.

3. **Focus on Relaxation:** Prior to anal play, engage in relaxation techniques such as deep breathing or gentle massages. A relaxed body is more receptive to anal stimulation.

4. **Gradual Size Increase:** Once comfortable with smaller toys, gradually increase the size. This can be done by using a series of toys that increase in diameter or length.

5. **Establish a Routine:** Consistency is key in anal training. Set aside regular time for training sessions, allowing the body to adapt over time.

6. **Communicate with Your Partner:** If training with a partner, maintain open lines of communication. Discuss comfort levels, boundaries, and desires to enhance the experience.

7. **Listen to Your Body:** Pay attention to your body's signals. If you experience pain or discomfort, take a step back and reassess your approach.

Examples of Anal Training Exercises

Here are a few exercises to incorporate into your anal training routine:

- **Finger Training:** Start with one well-lubricated finger. Gradually increase the number of fingers as comfort allows. Focus on slow, gentle movements to promote relaxation.

- **Toy Training:** Use a series of anal beads or a graduated set of anal plugs. Begin with the smallest size and work your way up, allowing your body to adjust to each new size.

- **Breath Control:** Practice deep, rhythmic breathing during anal play. Inhale deeply through the nose, hold for a moment, then exhale slowly. This can help alleviate anxiety and increase comfort.
- **Kegel Exercises:** Strengthening the pelvic floor muscles can enhance anal control and pleasure. Incorporate Kegel exercises into your routine to improve muscle tone and awareness.

Safety Considerations

Safety is paramount in anal training. Here are essential safety tips to keep in mind:

- **Use Body-Safe Materials:** Ensure that all toys and tools used for anal play are made from body-safe materials, such as silicone, glass, or stainless steel.
- **Avoid Cross-Contamination:** If switching between anal and vaginal play, always clean toys thoroughly to prevent the spread of bacteria.
- **Establish Safe Words:** If training with a partner, establish safe words to communicate comfort levels. This ensures that both partners can express their needs without hesitation.
- **Be Mindful of Hygiene:** Practice good hygiene before and after anal play. This includes washing hands and toys to minimize the risk of infection.

Conclusion

The art of anal training is a journey of exploration, trust, and pleasure. By understanding the principles of gradual adaptation, addressing common challenges, and implementing practical techniques, individuals can unlock new dimensions of pleasure. Remember that every journey is unique; take your time, communicate openly, and embrace the experience. The art of anal training is not just about physical sensations; it's about discovering the depths of your desires and expanding your sexual horizons.

Building Slave Skills through Consensual Anal Play

In the realm of BDSM, consensual anal play can serve as a powerful tool for building slave skills, fostering trust, and enhancing the dynamics between a Dominant and a submissive. This section will explore the theoretical underpinnings, practical applications, and challenges associated with developing these skills through anal play.

Theoretical Framework

The foundation of consensual anal play in BDSM is rooted in the principles of consent, trust, and communication. These elements are crucial in ensuring that both parties feel safe and respected throughout their exploration. According to the *RACK* (Risk Aware Consensual Kink) model, participants must be aware of the risks involved in anal play, including physical discomfort and emotional vulnerability. This awareness allows for informed decision-making and helps to establish a framework for safe exploration.

Skill Development

1. **Understanding the Role of Consent**   Before engaging in anal play, it is essential to have a clear and open dialogue about desires, limits, and boundaries. This conversation should include discussions about:

   + Personal comfort levels with anal play.
   + Specific activities that may be involved (e.g., anal penetration, fisting).
   + Safe words and signals to ensure immediate communication during play.

2. **Establishing Protocols**   Building slave skills often involves the establishment of protocols that govern behavior during play. These protocols can include:

   + Positioning: The submissive may be required to adopt specific positions that enhance vulnerability and submission.
   + Attitude: Expectations regarding the submissive's demeanor during play (e.g., maintaining eye contact, using honorifics).
   + Aftercare: Guidelines for post-play care that ensure emotional and physical well-being.

3. **Gradual Exposure**   For many submissives, especially those new to anal play, gradual exposure is key to building comfort and skill. This can be achieved through:

   + **Warm-up Techniques:** Start with external stimulation, such as anal massage or gentle pressure around the anal opening, to help the submissive relax.
   + **Progressive Penetration:** Use smaller toys or fingers to gradually increase the size and depth of penetration, allowing the submissive to acclimate to the sensations.

- **Feedback Loop:** Encourage the submissive to communicate openly about their comfort levels, adjusting techniques based on their responses.

Challenges and Solutions

1. **Addressing Discomfort**   Physical discomfort is a common challenge in anal play. To mitigate this, it is essential to:

    - Use ample lubrication to reduce friction.
    - Take breaks as needed, allowing the submissive to breathe and relax.
    - Incorporate breathing techniques to help manage discomfort and anxiety.

2. **Emotional Vulnerability**   Anal play can evoke a range of emotions, from pleasure to fear. To address emotional challenges:

    - Engage in pre-play discussions about feelings and fears.
    - Establish a debriefing period after play to discuss experiences and emotions.
    - Incorporate aftercare practices that provide comfort and reassurance.

3. **Navigating Societal Stigma**   Participants may encounter societal stigma surrounding anal play, which can affect their self-image and confidence. To combat this:

    - Foster a positive and affirming environment within the BDSM community.
    - Educate oneself and partners about the benefits of anal play, emphasizing its consensual nature.
    - Seek support from like-minded individuals who understand and accept diverse sexual practices.

Practical Examples

1. **Role-Playing Scenarios**   Engaging in role-playing can enhance the experience of consensual anal play. For instance, a Dominant might assume the role of a strict trainer, guiding the submissive through a series of tasks designed to build their anal skills. This could involve:

- Requiring the submissive to prepare themselves for anal play, emphasizing the importance of hygiene and relaxation.

- Using a variety of toys, gradually increasing in size and complexity, to help the submissive develop their comfort and skills.

2. Skill Challenges Incorporating skill challenges into anal play can be a fun and educational way to build slave skills. Examples include:

- Timing challenges where the submissive must maintain a specific position or hold a toy in place for a set duration.

- Sensation challenges that involve varying degrees of pressure or temperature during anal play, encouraging the submissive to articulate their pleasure and discomfort.

3. Feedback and Reflection After each session, the Dominant should encourage the submissive to provide feedback on their experience. This reflection can help identify areas for improvement and reinforce the skills learned during play. Questions to consider might include:

- What sensations were most pleasurable?

- Were there any moments of discomfort, and how can we address them in the future?

- How did the experience affect your emotional state?

Conclusion

Building slave skills through consensual anal play is a journey that requires patience, trust, and open communication. By understanding the theoretical framework, addressing challenges, and implementing practical techniques, participants can enhance their BDSM experiences while fostering deeper connections. Embracing this exploration not only enriches the dynamic between Dominant and submissive but also empowers individuals to discover new dimensions of pleasure and intimacy.

Establishing Protocols and Punishments

In the realm of BDSM, establishing clear protocols and punishments is crucial for ensuring a safe, consensual, and pleasurable experience for all parties involved. Protocols serve as guidelines that dictate behavior and expectations within the dynamic, while punishments can be employed as a means of reinforcing these protocols and enhancing the overall experience. This section explores the theory behind protocols and punishments, the potential challenges that may arise, and practical examples to illustrate their implementation.

Understanding Protocols

Protocols are structured rules or guidelines that define the relationship dynamics between partners. They can vary widely based on individual preferences, the nature of the relationship, and the specific activities involved. Establishing protocols serves several purposes:

- **Clarity:** Clear protocols provide a framework for behavior, reducing ambiguity and confusion during play.

- **Safety:** Protocols enhance safety by outlining boundaries and limits, ensuring that all parties are aware of what is acceptable and what is not.

- **Connection:** They foster a deeper connection between partners by creating a shared understanding of roles and responsibilities.

Types of Protocols

Protocols can be categorized into various types, including:

- **Behavioral Protocols:** Rules governing conduct, such as how a submissive should address their dominant partner or specific rituals to be performed before or after a scene.

- **Communication Protocols:** Guidelines for discussing desires, limits, and aftercare, ensuring that both partners feel heard and respected.

- **Safety Protocols:** Established safety measures, including the use of safe words, check-ins during play, and aftercare practices.

Establishing Effective Protocols

To establish effective protocols, consider the following steps:

1. **Open Dialogue:** Engage in open and honest conversations about desires, limits, and expectations. This dialogue should occur before any play begins.

2. **Mutual Agreement:** Ensure that all parties consent to the established protocols. This consent should be ongoing and can be revisited as dynamics evolve.

3. **Documentation:** Some partners find it helpful to document protocols in writing. This can serve as a reference and reinforce commitment to the established guidelines.

Understanding Punishments

Punishments in BDSM serve as a form of discipline that reinforces protocols and can heighten the intensity of the experience. It is essential to understand that punishments should never be abusive or harmful; they must always be consensual and agreed upon in advance.

Purpose of Punishments

The purposes of incorporating punishments into BDSM dynamics include:

- **Reinforcement:** Punishments reinforce the importance of adhering to protocols, helping partners remain accountable.

- **Behavior Modification:** They can be used to encourage specific behaviors or discourage unwanted actions.

- **Heightened Arousal:** For some, the anticipation and experience of punishment can enhance arousal and pleasure.

Types of Punishments

Punishments can take various forms, including:

- **Verbal Corrections:** A dominant partner may issue a verbal reprimand to remind the submissive of their protocols.

- **Physical Punishments:** This can include spanking, flogging, or other forms of impact play, always ensuring that safety measures are in place.

- **Time-Outs:** A submissive may be placed in a time-out to reflect on their behavior and the importance of the established protocols.

Challenges and Considerations

Establishing protocols and punishments can present challenges, including:

- **Miscommunication:** Clear communication is vital. Misunderstandings regarding protocols or punishments can lead to feelings of resentment or discomfort.

- **Emotional Responses:** Some individuals may experience strong emotional reactions to punishments. It is essential to engage in aftercare to address these feelings and reinforce trust.

- **Evolving Dynamics:** Relationships can change over time. Regularly revisiting and adjusting protocols and punishments ensures they remain relevant and consensual.

Practical Examples

Here are a few practical examples of protocols and punishments in action:

- **Example 1: Ritual Greeting Protocol** – A submissive may be required to greet their dominant partner in a specific manner, such as kneeling and expressing gratitude. Failure to do so may result in a verbal reprimand or a light spanking.

- **Example 2: Communication Protocol** – A couple may establish a protocol that requires the submissive to check in with their dominant partner before engaging in any solo play. If this protocol is breached, the submissive may face a temporary restriction on their playtime.

- **Example 3: Safety Protocol Violation** – If a submissive neglects to use a safe word during a scene, the dominant partner may impose a punishment, such as additional impact play, to reinforce the importance of safety and communication.

Conclusion

Establishing protocols and punishments is a fundamental aspect of BDSM dynamics that fosters safety, connection, and pleasure. By engaging in open communication, mutual consent, and ongoing negotiation, partners can create a fulfilling and empowering experience that honors their desires and boundaries. Remember, the key to successful protocols and punishments lies in trust, respect, and the shared commitment to enhance each other's pleasure in a consensual manner.

Exploring Boundaries and Limits

Communicating Desires and Negotiating Boundaries

Effective communication is the cornerstone of any intimate relationship, particularly when it comes to exploring anal play. Understanding how to articulate your desires and negotiate boundaries not only enhances the experience but also fosters a deeper connection between partners. This section will delve into the theory behind communication in sexual contexts, identify common challenges, and provide practical examples to facilitate open discussions about anal play.

Theoretical Framework

Communication in sexual relationships can be conceptualized through several key theories, including the **Social Exchange Theory** and **Relational Dialectics Theory**.

- **Social Exchange Theory** posits that individuals seek to maximize rewards and minimize costs in their interactions. This means that when discussing anal play, both partners should feel that the potential benefits (pleasure, intimacy, trust) outweigh any perceived risks (discomfort, emotional vulnerability).

- **Relational Dialectics Theory** suggests that relationships are characterized by ongoing tensions between opposing forces, such as autonomy and connection. In the context of anal play, partners may experience the tension between the desire for exploration and the need for safety and comfort. Addressing these dialectics openly can lead to healthier negotiations.

Identifying Common Problems

Despite the importance of communication, many individuals encounter obstacles when discussing sexual desires, particularly regarding anal play. Common issues include:

- **Fear of Judgment:** Individuals may worry about being judged for their desires, leading to reluctance in expressing themselves.

- **Misunderstandings:** Partners may interpret each other's signals differently, which can result in confusion or unmet expectations.

- **Lack of Vocabulary:** Some may struggle to find the right words to describe their desires, which can hinder effective communication.

Strategies for Effective Communication

To overcome these challenges, consider the following strategies:

- **Create a Safe Space:** Establish an environment where both partners feel comfortable discussing their desires without fear of judgment. This can be achieved by choosing a neutral location, setting aside dedicated time for the conversation, and emphasizing mutual respect.

- **Use "I" Statements:** Frame your desires using "I" statements to express feelings without placing blame. For example, instead of saying "You never want to try anal," you could say, "I feel excited about the idea of exploring anal play together."

- **Practice Active Listening:** Ensure that both partners have the opportunity to express their thoughts. Practice active listening by summarizing what your partner says and confirming your understanding before responding.

- **Discuss Limits and Boundaries:** Clearly articulate your personal limits and ask your partner about theirs. This can include physical boundaries, emotional readiness, and any specific activities that may be off-limits. For instance, "I am open to trying anal play, but I want to set a limit on how far we go tonight."

- **Utilize Visual Aids:** Sometimes, visual aids such as diagrams or videos can help clarify desires and techniques. Discussing these aids together can also serve as a conversation starter.

Examples of Communication Scenarios

To illustrate these strategies, here are a couple of examples:

- Scenario 1: Initial Discussion

    Partner A: "I've been thinking about trying anal play. I've read that it can be really pleasurable. What do you think?"

    Partner B: "I'm open to it, but I'm a bit nervous. Can we talk about what that might look like?"

    In this scenario, Partner A initiates the conversation, and Partner B responds with openness while expressing their concerns. This sets the stage for a deeper discussion about desires and boundaries.

- Scenario 2: Setting Boundaries

    Partner A: "I want to explore anal play, but I need to know that we can stop at any time if it becomes uncomfortable."

    Partner B: "Absolutely! Let's agree on a safe word we can use if we need to pause."

    Here, both partners express their desires while establishing a safety mechanism, demonstrating effective boundary negotiation.

Conclusion

Communicating desires and negotiating boundaries in anal play is not just about the act itself; it's about building trust, enhancing intimacy, and ensuring that both partners feel safe and respected. By employing effective communication strategies, individuals can navigate the complexities of their desires and create fulfilling experiences that honor their boundaries. Remember, the journey into anal pleasure is as much about the connection between partners as it is about the physical sensations. Embrace the conversation, and let it lead you toward deeper exploration and joy.

Open and Honest Communication

Open and honest communication is the cornerstone of any healthy sexual relationship, particularly when it comes to exploring anal play. This section will delve into the significance of transparent dialogue, the potential challenges that may arise, and practical strategies for fostering effective communication between partners.

The Importance of Communication

Effective communication serves multiple purposes in the realm of anal play:

1. **Establishing Trust**: Trust is fundamental in any intimate relationship, and it is especially critical when engaging in activities that may be perceived as taboo or that involve vulnerability. Open dialogue allows partners to express their feelings, fears, and desires, thereby building a foundation of trust.

2. **Setting Boundaries**: Each partner may have different comfort levels regarding anal play. Communicating these boundaries clearly helps prevent misunderstandings and ensures that both partners feel safe and respected. This can include discussing limits on penetration depth, types of stimulation, and the use of toys.

3. **Consent and Negotiation**: Consent is not a one-time agreement; it is an ongoing conversation. Partners should regularly check in with each other, especially as they explore new techniques or activities. This ongoing negotiation allows for a more fluid and responsive sexual experience.

4. **Addressing Concerns**: Open communication provides a platform for partners to voice any concerns they may have, whether related to physical discomfort, emotional responses, or external pressures. Addressing these issues proactively can enhance the overall experience and strengthen the emotional bond between partners.

Challenges to Communication

Despite its importance, open communication can be challenging for many couples. Some common barriers include:

- **Fear of Judgment**: Partners may worry about being judged for their desires or fears. This fear can inhibit honest expression and create a barrier to exploring anal play.
- **Cultural and Societal Influences**: Societal stigma surrounding anal play can lead to feelings of shame or embarrassment. Partners may have internalized these messages, making it difficult to discuss their interests openly.
- **Lack of Knowledge**: If one or both partners are unfamiliar with anal anatomy or techniques, they may feel unsure about how to communicate their needs effectively. This lack of knowledge can lead to confusion and frustration.

Strategies for Effective Communication

To overcome these barriers, consider the following strategies for fostering open and honest communication:

1. **Create a Safe Space**: Establish a non-judgmental environment where both partners feel comfortable sharing their thoughts and feelings. This can be achieved by choosing a neutral location, such as a quiet room, and setting aside dedicated time for discussion.

2. **Use "I" Statements**: Encourage the use of "I" statements to express feelings and needs without placing blame. For example, saying "I feel anxious about trying anal play" is more constructive than "You make me feel anxious about anal play."

3. **Practice Active Listening**: Listening is just as important as speaking. Ensure that both partners have the opportunity to share their thoughts and feelings without interruption. Reflect back what you hear to confirm understanding, such as, "So what I hear you saying is…"

4. **Check-In Regularly**: Make it a habit to check in with each other before, during, and after anal play. This can be as simple as asking, "How are you feeling about this?" or "Is there anything you want to change?" Regular check-ins help maintain an open dialogue.

5. **Educate Together**: Consider exploring resources together, such as books, workshops, or online courses about anal play. Learning together can enhance understanding and provide common ground for discussion.

6. **Use Humor**: Sometimes, humor can help break the ice and alleviate tension. Sharing a laugh about the awkwardness of discussing anal play can create a more relaxed atmosphere.

Examples of Communication Scenarios

To illustrate the importance of open communication in anal play, consider the following scenarios:

- **Scenario 1**: Before engaging in anal play, Partner A expresses a desire to try anal penetration. Partner B feels apprehensive but does not want to disappoint Partner A. Instead of suppressing their feelings, Partner B shares their concerns about discomfort and the need for gradual exploration. This open dialogue allows them to agree on starting with external stimulation before progressing.

- **Scenario 2**: During a session, Partner A experiences discomfort during anal penetration. Instead of continuing in silence, Partner A communicates their feelings, saying, "I'm feeling a bit uncomfortable right now." Partner B responds by

EXPLORING BOUNDARIES AND LIMITS 167

pausing and asking what adjustments can be made to enhance comfort, demonstrating the importance of responsiveness and adaptability.

Conclusion

In conclusion, open and honest communication is vital for a fulfilling and pleasurable anal play experience. By establishing trust, setting clear boundaries, and addressing concerns proactively, partners can navigate the complexities of anal play with confidence and enthusiasm. Ultimately, fostering an environment of transparency and respect not only enhances the sexual experience but also strengthens the emotional bond between partners, paving the way for deeper intimacy and exploration.

Establishing Safe Words and Signals

In any form of sexual exploration, especially in anal play and BDSM contexts, establishing safe words and signals is crucial for ensuring that all parties feel secure and respected. Safe words serve as a clear and unambiguous method of communication, allowing participants to express their comfort levels and boundaries without ambiguity. This section will delve into the importance of safe words and signals, how to choose them, and the best practices for implementing them in your intimate experiences.

The Importance of Safe Words

Safe words are essential tools for maintaining safety and consent during sexual activities. They provide a way to communicate discomfort or the need to pause or stop the activity altogether. The importance of safe words can be understood through several key principles:

- **Clear Communication:** Safe words eliminate ambiguity. Unlike regular language, which can be misinterpreted during heightened states of arousal, a safe word is pre-agreed upon and understood by all parties.

- **Empowerment:** Establishing a safe word empowers individuals to take control of their experience. It reinforces the notion that everyone involved has the right to change their mind at any point.

- **Trust Building:** The act of agreeing on safe words fosters trust between partners. It demonstrates a commitment to each other's well-being and comfort.

- **Safety Net:** In the context of BDSM, where power dynamics may shift, safe words act as a safety net, ensuring that all participants can engage in activities without fear of crossing personal boundaries.

Choosing Safe Words

When selecting safe words, it is important to choose terms that are easy to remember, distinct, and unlikely to be used in the heat of the moment. Here are some guidelines for choosing effective safe words:

- **Simplicity:** Choose a word that is simple and easy to pronounce. Common choices include "red" for stop, "yellow" for slow down, and "green" for continue.

- **Unambiguous:** The chosen word should not be something that might be confused with other terms used during play. For example, using "no" as a safe word can be problematic, as it may be used in a playful context.

- **Memorable:** Select a word that is easy to remember. Avoid complex phrases or obscure references that may not come to mind during intense moments.

- **Personal Preference:** Encourage each participant to choose a word that resonates with them personally. This could be a favorite color, an animal, or any other term that feels comfortable.

Implementing Safe Words in Practice

Once safe words have been established, it is crucial to implement them effectively during play. Here are some best practices for using safe words:

- **Pre-Play Discussion:** Before engaging in any sexual activity, have an open conversation about the safe words and signals. Ensure everyone understands their meanings and agrees to respect them.

- **Regular Check-Ins:** During play, it is beneficial to have regular check-ins with each other. This can be verbal or non-verbal. For example, a simple thumbs up or down can help gauge comfort levels.

- **Immediate Response:** If a safe word is spoken, all activity should cease immediately. It is essential to respect the request without question or hesitation.

- **Aftercare:** After the activity, engage in aftercare to discuss the experience. This includes checking in on emotional and physical well-being and addressing any feelings that may have arisen during play.

Signals for Non-Verbal Communication

In situations where verbal communication may be difficult, such as during intense moments of pleasure or if one partner is gagged, establishing non-verbal signals is equally important. These signals can include:

- **Hand Signals:** Agree on specific hand gestures that signify different levels of comfort or the need to stop. For example, holding up a hand with fingers spread could mean "stop," while a fist might indicate "I'm okay."

- **Tapping:** A light tap on the arm or leg can serve as a signal to pause or check in. This method is particularly effective in scenarios where verbal communication is hindered.

- **Props:** Some individuals may choose to use physical objects, such as a bell or a specific item that can be dropped, to indicate the need to stop or slow down.

Examples of Safe Words and Signals

To illustrate the concepts discussed, here are a few examples of effective safe words and non-verbal signals:

- **Safe Words:**

    - "Red" for stop
    - "Yellow" for slow down or check-in
    - "Green" for continue

- **Non-Verbal Signals:**

    - Thumbs up for "I'm good"
    - Thumbs down for "Stop"
    - A light squeeze of the hand for "Check-in"

Conclusion

Establishing safe words and signals is a fundamental aspect of engaging in anal play and BDSM activities. They enhance communication, empower individuals, and foster trust, ensuring that all participants can explore their desires safely and consensually. By choosing effective safe words, implementing them thoughtfully, and considering non-verbal signals, partners can create a secure environment that encourages exploration and pleasure. Remember, the key to a fulfilling sexual experience lies in open communication and mutual respect.

Respecting Personal Boundaries and Limits

In the realm of anal play, respecting personal boundaries and limits is not merely a courtesy; it is the cornerstone of a safe and pleasurable experience. Every participant in anal play has unique comfort levels, desires, and boundaries that must be understood and honored. This section delves into the importance of boundaries, how to communicate them effectively, and the consequences of neglecting this vital aspect of sexual exploration.

Understanding Boundaries

Personal boundaries refer to the physical, emotional, and psychological limits that individuals establish to protect themselves in intimate situations. These boundaries can vary significantly between individuals and can be influenced by past experiences, cultural backgrounds, and personal beliefs. In anal play, boundaries might include:

- **Physical Boundaries:** These involve what types of touch, penetration, or stimulation are acceptable. For example, one partner may be comfortable with anal fingering but not with penetration using toys or a penis.
- **Emotional Boundaries:** These relate to how a person feels about certain actions and the emotional implications of those actions. Some might find that certain types of anal play evoke feelings of vulnerability or anxiety.
- **Psychological Boundaries:** These encompass mental and emotional triggers that could lead to discomfort or distress. Understanding triggers is crucial for maintaining a safe space.

Communicating Boundaries

Effective communication is essential for respecting personal boundaries. Here are some strategies to facilitate open dialogue about limits:

1. **Pre-Play Discussions:** Before engaging in anal play, partners should have an open and honest conversation about their boundaries. This discussion should cover what is off-limits, what is desired, and any fears or concerns.

2. **Use of Safe Words:** Establishing a safe word is a powerful tool for maintaining boundaries during play. A safe word should be easy to remember and distinctly different from other words used during play. For example, using "red" to indicate a need to stop immediately can be effective.

3. **Check-Ins:** During anal play, it's important to check in with your partner regularly. Simple questions like "How are you feeling?" or "Is this okay?" can help ensure that both partners feel safe and respected.

4. **Non-Verbal Signals:** In addition to verbal communication, non-verbal cues can be crucial. Partners should be attuned to body language and physical reactions, which can indicate discomfort or pleasure.

Consequences of Ignoring Boundaries

Neglecting to respect personal boundaries can lead to a range of negative outcomes, including:

- **Physical Injury:** Ignoring limits can result in physical harm, including tearing, pain, or other injuries that can lead to long-term discomfort.

- **Emotional Distress:** Disregarding emotional boundaries can lead to feelings of betrayal, anxiety, or trauma. This can have lasting effects on a person's relationship with intimacy and trust.

- **Breakdown of Trust:** Trust is foundational in any intimate relationship. Violating boundaries can erode trust, making future encounters fraught with tension and apprehension.

Examples of Boundary Setting

To illustrate the importance of respecting personal boundaries, consider the following scenarios:

- **Scenario 1:** Partner A expresses discomfort with anal penetration but is open to anal fingering. Partner B respects this boundary and focuses solely on the agreed-upon activity, enhancing trust and intimacy.

- **Scenario 2:** During a session, Partner A uses a safe word to indicate discomfort. Partner B immediately stops the activity, demonstrating respect for boundaries and prioritizing Partner A's well-being.

- **Scenario 3:** Partner A and Partner B discuss their limits before engaging in anal play, establishing clear expectations. This proactive approach leads to a more enjoyable experience for both parties.

Conclusion

Respecting personal boundaries and limits is not only essential for safe anal play but also for fostering trust, intimacy, and mutual enjoyment. By engaging in open communication, establishing safe words, and being attentive to each other's needs, partners can create a fulfilling and pleasurable anal experience. Remember, boundaries are not barriers; they are the framework within which pleasure can thrive.

Debriefing and Aftercare

Aftercare is an essential component of any intimate experience, particularly in the realm of anal play where emotional and physical boundaries can be tested. This section will explore the importance of debriefing and aftercare, providing theoretical insights, potential challenges, and practical examples to enhance the overall experience of anal enthusiasts.

The Importance of Aftercare

Aftercare refers to the time spent caring for and nurturing one another after an intense experience, whether sexual or emotional. This practice serves several purposes:

- **Emotional Reconnection**: After engaging in anal play, partners may feel vulnerable. Aftercare provides an opportunity to reconnect emotionally, reinforcing intimacy and trust.

- **Physical Comfort**: Anal play can sometimes lead to discomfort or physical sensations that linger after the act. Aftercare allows for addressing these physical needs through soothing touch, communication, or even medical attention if necessary.

- **Processing the Experience**: Engaging in debriefing allows partners to share their feelings about the experience, discuss what they enjoyed, what they found challenging, and how they can improve future encounters.

Theoretical Framework

The theory of aftercare can be rooted in several psychological principles:

- **Attachment Theory**: This theory posits that secure attachments lead to healthier relationships. Aftercare can strengthen these attachments, as partners demonstrate care and concern for each other's well-being.

- **Polyvagal Theory**: This theory emphasizes the role of the vagus nerve in emotional regulation. Aftercare can help partners transition from heightened arousal states to a more calm and connected state, promoting safety and security.

- **Trauma-Informed Care**: Understanding that individuals may have past traumas that affect their responses during intimate moments can guide partners in providing sensitive aftercare that respects each other's boundaries and emotional needs.

Common Problems in Aftercare

While aftercare is crucial, it can sometimes present challenges. Here are a few common issues and how to address them:

- **Miscommunication**: Partners may have different expectations about what aftercare entails. It is essential to communicate openly about needs and desires regarding aftercare practices.

- **Emotional Disconnection**: Some individuals may feel emotionally drained or distant after intense experiences. It is important to check in with one another, allowing space for feelings to surface without judgment.

- **Physical Discomfort**: Anal play can lead to soreness or discomfort. Partners should discuss any physical sensations openly, allowing for adjustments in future experiences and ensuring that aftercare includes physical comfort measures, such as warm baths or soothing ointments.

Practical Examples of Aftercare

Here are some practical suggestions for aftercare following anal play:

1. **Physical Touch**: Cuddling, gentle massages, or skin-to-skin contact can help reinforce feelings of safety and intimacy. For example, a partner might run their fingers along the other's back, providing a calming effect.

2. **Hydration and Nutrition**: Offering water, herbal tea, or light snacks can help partners feel nurtured and cared for. This is especially important if any physical exertion occurred during play.

3. **Verbal Affirmations**: Sharing positive affirmations about the experience can enhance emotional connection. Phrases like "I really enjoyed that" or "I appreciate how you took care of me" can reinforce trust.

4. **Check-ins**: Partners should engage in a debriefing conversation. Questions such as "What did you enjoy most?" or "Is there anything you would like to try differently next time?" can facilitate open communication.

5. **Creating a Relaxing Environment**: Aftercare can be enhanced by creating a soothing atmosphere with dim lighting, soft music, or aromatherapy. This environment can promote relaxation and emotional safety.

Conclusion

Debriefing and aftercare are vital components of anal play that enhance the overall experience for both partners. By prioritizing emotional and physical care, partners can deepen their connection, address any concerns, and ensure that both individuals feel valued and respected. Embracing the practice of aftercare not only fosters intimacy but also empowers individuals to explore their desires safely and joyfully.

Ultimately, aftercare is about embracing vulnerability, celebrating shared experiences, and nurturing the bond that exists between partners. As you continue your journey into anal play, remember that the moments spent in aftercare can be just as pleasurable and rewarding as the acts themselves.

EXPLORING BOUNDARIES AND LIMITS

Anal Play in Non-Monogamous Relationships

Navigating Anal Play in Open Relationships

In the landscape of modern sexuality, open relationships offer a unique framework for exploring desires and pleasures that may not be fully realized within traditional monogamous settings. This section will delve into the intricacies of navigating anal play specifically within open relationships, addressing the complexities of trust, communication, and pleasure.

Understanding Open Relationships

Open relationships can take various forms, ranging from swinging to polyamory. Each structure has its own rules and dynamics, but the core principle remains the same: multiple consensual sexual or romantic relationships. This freedom can enrich sexual experiences, including anal play, by introducing new partners and perspectives. However, it also requires a strong foundation of trust and communication to ensure that all parties feel secure and respected.

Establishing Clear Communication

Effective communication is the cornerstone of successful anal play in open relationships. Partners must engage in open dialogues about their desires, boundaries, and concerns. This can involve discussing:

- **Desires and Interests:** What specific forms of anal play are you and your partner interested in exploring with others? Are there specific fantasies or techniques that excite you?
- **Boundaries:** What are the non-negotiables in your relationship? Establishing clear boundaries around anal play, such as who can participate and what activities are acceptable, is crucial.
- **Health and Safety:** Discussing safe sex practices, including the use of condoms and dental dams, is essential to prevent the transmission of sexually transmitted infections (STIs).

Navigating Jealousy and Insecurity

Jealousy can be a significant challenge in open relationships, particularly when it comes to intimate activities like anal play. Here are strategies to address these feelings:

- **Acknowledge Feelings:** Recognize that feelings of jealousy or insecurity are natural. Instead of suppressing these emotions, discuss them openly with your partner.

- **Reassurance:** Provide each other with reassurance about your commitment and love. Verbal affirmations can help mitigate feelings of inadequacy or fear.

- **Regular Check-Ins:** Schedule regular discussions to assess how each partner is feeling about the dynamics of the open relationship. This allows for adjustments to be made as necessary.

Creating a Safe Space for Exploration

When engaging in anal play with new partners, creating a safe and comfortable environment is vital. Here are some tips:

- **Choose the Right Setting:** Select a private and comfortable space where all parties feel at ease. This might be someone's home or a designated space that allows for intimacy.

- **Use Safe Words:** Establish safe words or signals that can be used to pause or stop the activity if anyone feels uncomfortable. This ensures that everyone feels empowered to communicate their needs.

- **Establish Aftercare:** Aftercare is essential, especially after intense experiences like anal play. Discuss what aftercare looks like for each partner, whether it involves cuddling, talking, or simply spending quiet time together.

Integrating New Partners into Anal Play

When introducing new partners into your anal play experiences, consider the following:

- **Consent:** Ensure that all parties involved have consented to the activities. Consent must be informed, enthusiastic, and ongoing.

- **Building Trust:** Take the time to build rapport with new partners. Trust is essential for a pleasurable experience, especially in anal play, which requires vulnerability.

- **Discussing Preferences:** Each partner may have different preferences and comfort levels regarding anal play. Discuss these openly to find common ground.

Example Scenarios

To illustrate the concepts discussed, consider the following scenarios:

- **Scenario 1:** Alex and Jamie are in an open relationship and decide to explore anal play with a new partner, Taylor. They have a pre-play discussion where they outline their desires, establish boundaries, and agree on safe words. Afterward, they engage in anal play, ensuring that everyone feels comfortable and respected. They follow up with aftercare to reinforce their bond.

- **Scenario 2:** Morgan feels insecure about their partner, Casey, exploring anal play with others. They communicate their feelings, leading to a deeper understanding of each other's needs. Casey reassures Morgan of their commitment, and they establish regular check-ins to maintain open communication.

Conclusion

Navigating anal play in open relationships can be a rewarding and fulfilling experience when approached with care and consideration. By prioritizing communication, establishing trust, and respecting boundaries, partners can explore their desires in a safe and consensual manner. Embracing the complexities of open relationships can lead to profound personal growth and deeper connections with oneself and others. As you embark on this journey, remember that the key to success lies in open dialogue, mutual respect, and a commitment to pleasure for all involved.

Maintaining Trust and Boundaries with Multiple Partners

Navigating anal play within non-monogamous relationships can be both exhilarating and complex. The key to a fulfilling experience lies in establishing trust and clear boundaries among all partners involved. This section explores the principles of maintaining trust and boundaries in a multi-partner context, highlighting the importance of communication, consent, and emotional safety.

The Importance of Communication

Effective communication is the cornerstone of any successful relationship, especially in non-monogamous arrangements. It is essential to openly discuss desires, boundaries, and expectations with each partner. This communication should be ongoing and adaptable, as feelings and circumstances may change over time.

- **Initial Conversations:** At the outset of any relationship, especially in a polyamorous context, partners should engage in deep discussions about their sexual preferences, including anal play. Questions to consider include:

    - What are your boundaries regarding anal play with other partners?
    - How do you feel about sharing intimate experiences with multiple partners?
    - What are your safe words, and how do you prefer to communicate during play?

- **Regular Check-Ins:** Schedule regular check-ins to discuss feelings and experiences. This can help address any discomfort or jealousy that may arise and ensure that all partners feel heard and respected.

Setting Clear Boundaries

Boundaries are essential for maintaining trust and emotional safety. Each partner should articulate their personal limits and understand those of others. Consider the following strategies for establishing and respecting boundaries:

- **Define Personal Limits:** Each partner should identify what they are comfortable with regarding anal play. This includes discussing:

    - Types of anal activities (e.g., penetration, fisting, use of toys)
    - Emotional boundaries (e.g., how intimacy is shared)
    - Physical boundaries (e.g., hygiene practices, safe sex)

- **Use of Safe Words:** Establish safe words that can be used by any partner to pause or stop any activity. This creates a safety net that allows for immediate communication of discomfort.

- **Respecting Boundaries:** It is vital to respect the boundaries set by each partner. Violating these boundaries can lead to feelings of betrayal and mistrust. If a partner expresses discomfort, it is essential to address their concerns without judgment.

Building Trust Among Partners

Trust is built through consistent actions and transparency. Here are some strategies to foster trust in a multi-partner environment:

- **Transparency:** Be open about your sexual activities with other partners. This does not mean sharing every detail, but being honest about what you are doing can prevent misunderstandings and feelings of betrayal.

- **Emotional Support:** Provide emotional support to each partner. This includes being there for them during vulnerable moments and validating their feelings. Building emotional intimacy can enhance trust significantly.

- **Reassurance:** Regularly reassure partners of their importance in your life. Affirmations can help alleviate insecurities that may arise in a non-monogamous setup.

Addressing Jealousy and Insecurity

Jealousy is a common challenge in non-monogamous relationships. It is essential to recognize and address these feelings constructively:

- **Acknowledge Feelings:** Encourage partners to express feelings of jealousy or insecurity. Acknowledging these emotions without judgment can help partners feel validated and understood.

- **Discuss Triggers:** Identify what specifically triggers feelings of jealousy. This could be certain behaviors, situations, or even specific partners. Open discussions can lead to better understanding and solutions.

- **Revisit Agreements:** If jealousy arises, revisit the agreements made regarding boundaries and communication. This can help partners realign and adjust to each other's needs.

Example Scenario

Consider a situation where Partner A engages in anal play with Partner B while also having a relationship with Partner C. Partner A should communicate with both partners about their experiences, ensuring that Partner C is comfortable with the activities taking place with Partner B.

If Partner C expresses discomfort or jealousy about Partner A's activities, it is crucial for Partner A to listen, validate those feelings, and discuss how they can address the concerns together. They might agree to set specific boundaries regarding anal play with other partners or establish more frequent check-ins to foster trust.

Conclusion

Maintaining trust and boundaries in non-monogamous relationships, particularly when engaging in anal play, requires open communication, respect for personal limits, and ongoing emotional support. By fostering a safe environment where all partners feel heard and valued, you can create a fulfilling and pleasurable experience that honors everyone's desires and boundaries. Remember, the journey of exploration is as important as the destination, and the connections you build along the way will enhance your experiences together.

Pleasure and Connection in Polyamorous Anal Play

In the realm of polyamorous relationships, anal play can serve as a powerful tool for enhancing pleasure and deepening connections among partners. The dynamics of multiple relationships introduce unique opportunities for exploration, intimacy, and shared experiences. However, navigating these waters requires clear communication, trust, and a mutual understanding of desires and boundaries.

Understanding Polyamory and Anal Play

Polyamory is defined as engaging in multiple consensual romantic or sexual relationships simultaneously. This lifestyle emphasizes open communication and consent, which are crucial when introducing anal play into the mix. The multifaceted nature of polyamorous relationships can amplify the pleasure derived from anal play, as partners may bring diverse techniques, preferences, and emotional connections to the experience.

Theoretical Framework

The theory of *relational dialectics* posits that relationships are characterized by ongoing tensions between opposing forces, such as autonomy and connection. In polyamorous dynamics, individuals may experience the desire for personal agency while simultaneously yearning for deeper intimacy with multiple partners. Anal play can bridge this gap by fostering a sense of connection through shared vulnerability and pleasure.

Building Trust and Communication

To ensure a fulfilling experience, partners must establish a foundation of trust and open communication. Here are key strategies to facilitate this process:

- **Pre-Play Discussions:** Prior to engaging in anal play, partners should discuss their desires, boundaries, and any specific concerns. This conversation should include topics such as comfort levels with anal play, preferred techniques, and any past experiences that may influence the current encounter.

- **Establishing Safe Words:** Safe words are essential in any sexual activity, but they hold particular significance in anal play due to its potential for discomfort. Establishing a clear and mutually agreed-upon safe word can help partners navigate their experiences safely and confidently.

- **Post-Play Debriefing:** After engaging in anal play, partners should take the time to discuss their experiences. This debriefing allows individuals to express what they enjoyed, any discomfort they felt, and how the experience affected their connection. This practice not only enhances future encounters but also strengthens emotional bonds.

Exploring Pleasure in a Polyamorous Context

Anal play can provide unique pleasure experiences that vary between partners. Here are some ways to explore pleasure and connection through anal play in polyamorous relationships:

- **Variety of Techniques:** Each partner may have different preferences and techniques that enhance pleasure. For example, one partner may enjoy gentle anal stimulation, while another may prefer more intense sensations. Mixing these techniques can create a richer experience for everyone involved.

- **Shared Experiences:** Engaging in anal play as a group can foster a sense of community and shared intimacy. Consider scenarios where partners take turns stimulating one another, creating a rhythm that enhances collective pleasure. This can be particularly powerful during group play sessions or intimate gatherings.

- **Role Reversal:** In polyamorous relationships, partners may have the opportunity to explore different roles during anal play. For instance, a partner who typically takes on a submissive role may wish to explore dominance, or vice versa. This role reversal can deepen emotional connections and expand the boundaries of pleasure.

Potential Challenges

While anal play can enhance pleasure and connection, it is not without challenges. Here are some common issues that may arise and strategies to address them:

- **Jealousy and Insecurity:** In polyamorous relationships, feelings of jealousy may surface, particularly when engaging in intimate acts like anal play. Addressing these feelings openly can help partners navigate their emotions and reinforce trust.

- **Differing Comfort Levels:** Not all partners may feel comfortable with anal play. It is crucial to respect each individual's boundaries and preferences. Engaging in discussions about comfort levels can help partners find alternative ways to connect and explore pleasure together.

- **Logistical Considerations:** Coordinating anal play with multiple partners can present logistical challenges, such as finding suitable times and spaces. Open communication about scheduling and preferences can help mitigate these issues and ensure that everyone involved feels valued and included.

Conclusion

Incorporating anal play into polyamorous relationships can enhance pleasure and deepen connections among partners. By fostering open communication, establishing trust, and exploring diverse techniques, individuals can create a fulfilling and enriching sexual experience. Embracing the unique dynamics of polyamory allows partners to celebrate their desires and cultivate a deeper understanding of one another through the shared exploration of anal pleasure.

As you embark on this journey, remember that the key to unlocking pleasure and connection lies in communication, consent, and the willingness to explore the depths of your desires together. Embrace the adventure and enjoy the myriad of possibilities that polyamorous anal play has to offer.

Overcoming Challenges and Setbacks

Dealing with Pain and Discomfort

Engaging in anal play can sometimes lead to experiences of pain and discomfort, which can be disheartening for both novices and seasoned enthusiasts. Understanding the causes of such sensations and knowing how to address them is crucial for a pleasurable and fulfilling experience. This section aims to equip readers with strategies to manage pain and discomfort effectively.

Understanding Pain in Anal Play

Pain during anal play can arise from various factors, including physical, psychological, and emotional aspects. Recognizing the source of discomfort is the first step in addressing it.

Physical Causes

- **Tension and Anxiety:** The body's natural response to anxiety is muscle tension, particularly in the pelvic floor. This tension can lead to discomfort during penetration.

- **Insufficient Lubrication:** The anus does not produce its own lubrication, making it essential to use adequate amounts of lubricant to facilitate smooth insertion and reduce friction.

- **Inadequate Preparation:** Rushing into anal play without proper preparation can lead to pain. This includes physical preparation, such as relaxation and stretching.

- **Health Conditions:** Certain medical conditions, such as hemorrhoids, anal fissures, or infections, can cause significant discomfort during anal play. It is vital to consult a healthcare professional if any underlying health issues are suspected.

Psychological Causes

- **Fear and Anticipation:** Fear of pain can create a psychological barrier that heightens sensitivity to discomfort. This anticipatory anxiety can manifest physically, leading to a cycle of tension and pain.

- **Negative Past Experiences:** Previous painful experiences can influence current encounters, making individuals more apprehensive and sensitive to discomfort.

Strategies for Managing Pain and Discomfort

To enhance the experience of anal play and minimize discomfort, consider implementing the following strategies:

1. Communication   Open and honest communication with your partner is essential. Discuss any fears, boundaries, and preferences before engaging in anal play. Establishing a safe word or signal can help both partners feel secure and in control.

2. Relaxation Techniques   Incorporating relaxation techniques can help alleviate tension. Consider the following methods:

- **Deep Breathing:** Practice deep, slow breaths to calm the mind and body. Inhale deeply through the nose, hold for a moment, and exhale slowly through the mouth.

- **Progressive Muscle Relaxation:** Gradually tense and then relax different muscle groups in the body, focusing on the pelvic floor. This technique can help reduce overall tension.

- **Warm Baths:** Taking a warm bath before engaging in anal play can relax the muscles and ease anxiety.

3. Adequate Lubrication   Using a high-quality lubricant is crucial for anal play. Water-based or silicone-based lubricants are recommended. Apply a generous amount before and during penetration to reduce friction and enhance comfort.

4. Gradual Insertion   Start with smaller toys or fingers and gradually increase size and depth. This gradual approach allows the body to adjust and reduces the likelihood of discomfort.

5. Use of Relaxation Tools   Consider using anal training kits, which include a range of toys designed to help individuals acclimate to anal play. These kits typically feature progressively larger sizes and can assist in easing into anal experiences.

6. Addressing Health Issues If pain persists despite implementing the above strategies, it is crucial to seek professional medical advice. Conditions such as hemorrhoids or anal fissures may require treatment before resuming anal play.

When to Stop

Listening to your body is paramount. If you experience sharp, severe pain or discomfort that does not subside, it is essential to stop immediately. Pain is a signal that something may not be right, and ignoring it can lead to injury or lasting damage.

1. Recognizing Pain Levels Understanding the difference between discomfort and pain is vital. Discomfort can often be a part of the experience as the body adjusts, but sharp or intense pain is not normal.

2. Aftercare Aftercare is an essential component of any sexual experience, particularly after anal play. Engage in soothing activities such as cuddling, gentle touch, or discussing the experience. This practice helps reinforce trust and intimacy between partners.

Conclusion

Dealing with pain and discomfort during anal play is a common concern that can be managed through awareness, communication, and proper techniques. By understanding the causes of discomfort and implementing strategies to address them, individuals can enhance their anal experiences and embrace the pleasure that comes with exploration. Remember, the journey towards anal pleasure is personal and should be approached with care, patience, and respect for oneself and one's partner.

Addressing Emotional and Psychological Challenges

Engaging in anal play can evoke a variety of emotional and psychological responses, stemming from societal conditioning, personal experiences, and individual expectations. Understanding and addressing these challenges is crucial for a fulfilling and positive sexual experience. This section explores common emotional hurdles, relevant theories, and practical strategies to navigate these complexities.

Understanding Emotional Responses

Emotional responses to anal play can range from excitement and pleasure to anxiety and fear. These reactions may be influenced by several factors, including:

- **Cultural Stigma:** Societal norms often label anal play as taboo, leading to feelings of shame or guilt. This stigma can create internal conflict, making it challenging for individuals to embrace their desires.

- **Past Experiences:** Previous negative experiences, whether related to anal play or general sexual encounters, can lead to anxiety or fear surrounding anal activities. These feelings may manifest as apprehension or reluctance to engage in anal play.

- **Expectations and Pressure:** The desire to meet perceived standards of pleasure or performance can create anxiety. Individuals may feel pressured to achieve specific outcomes, which can detract from the enjoyment of the experience.

Theoretical Frameworks

Several psychological theories can help in understanding the emotional challenges related to anal play:

- **Cognitive Behavioral Theory (CBT):** This theory posits that our thoughts influence our feelings and behaviors. Negative thoughts about anal play, such as fear of pain or judgment, can lead to anxiety. CBT techniques can help individuals identify and reframe these thoughts to foster a more positive mindset.

- **Attachment Theory:** This theory explores how early relationships with caregivers shape our emotional responses and interpersonal dynamics. Individuals with insecure attachment styles may struggle with trust and intimacy, which can complicate anal play experiences.

- **Mindfulness-Based Approaches:** Mindfulness encourages present-moment awareness and acceptance of one's feelings without judgment. Practicing mindfulness can help individuals acknowledge and process their emotions related to anal play, reducing anxiety and enhancing pleasure.

Common Psychological Challenges

1. **Anxiety and Fear:** Many individuals experience anxiety about anal play, fearing pain, embarrassment, or judgment. This anxiety can create a cycle of avoidance, where the fear of engaging in anal play prevents individuals from exploring their desires.

$$\text{Anxiety} = f(\text{Fear of Pain, Fear of Judgment, Previous Experiences}) \quad (30)$$

Example: A person may feel anxious about trying anal play due to a past experience where they felt discomfort or were ridiculed by a partner. This fear can prevent them from exploring anal pleasure in future relationships.

2. **Shame and Guilt:** Cultural messages often instill feelings of shame or guilt around anal play. These emotions can be deeply rooted and may require conscious effort to address.

$$\text{Shame} = g(\text{Cultural Norms, Personal Beliefs, Peer Influence}) \quad (31)$$

Example: An individual raised in a conservative environment may struggle with feelings of guilt when considering anal play, fearing judgment from peers or family.

3. **Difficulty with Trust and Intimacy:** Engaging in anal play often requires a high level of trust and intimacy between partners. Individuals who have experienced betrayal or emotional trauma may find it challenging to fully engage in anal play.

$$\text{Trust Issues} = h(\text{Past Trauma, Attachment Style, Communication Skills}) \quad (32)$$

Example: A person who has previously experienced infidelity may find it difficult to trust their partner during anal play, leading to feelings of insecurity and anxiety.

Strategies for Addressing Emotional Challenges

1. **Open Communication:** Establishing open lines of communication with partners is essential. Discussing fears, desires, and boundaries can help alleviate anxiety and build trust.

- **Use "I" Statements:** Express feelings using "I" statements to avoid placing blame. For example, "I feel anxious about trying anal play because I'm afraid of pain."

- **Active Listening:** Practice active listening to ensure both partners feel heard and validated in their feelings.

2. **Educate Yourself:** Knowledge can empower individuals to overcome fear and anxiety. Understanding the anatomy, safety precautions, and techniques can help demystify anal play.

- **Read Books and Articles:** Explore literature that discusses anal play, anatomy, and techniques.
- **Attend Workshops or Classes:** Participating in educational workshops can provide practical insights and foster a sense of community.

3. **Practice Mindfulness and Relaxation Techniques:** Incorporating mindfulness practices can help individuals manage anxiety and enhance their connection to their bodies.

- **Deep Breathing Exercises:** Practice deep breathing before and during anal play to promote relaxation.
- **Meditation:** Engage in meditation to cultivate present-moment awareness and reduce anxiety.

4. **Gradual Exposure:** Start with less intense forms of anal play to build comfort and confidence. Gradually increasing the intensity can help individuals acclimate to the experience.

- **Begin with External Stimulation:** Explore anal play through external stimulation before progressing to penetration.
- **Use Smaller Toys:** Incorporate smaller anal toys to ease into the experience gradually.

5. **Seek Professional Support:** If emotional challenges persist, consider seeking support from a therapist or counselor specializing in sexual health. Professional guidance can provide valuable insights and coping strategies.

- **Therapeutic Techniques:** Cognitive-behavioral therapy (CBT) can help address negative thought patterns and anxiety.
- **Support Groups:** Joining support groups can foster a sense of community and shared experiences.

Conclusion

Addressing emotional and psychological challenges related to anal play is a vital aspect of the journey toward sexual empowerment. By understanding the underlying factors contributing to anxiety, shame, and trust issues, individuals can develop effective strategies to navigate these complexities. Open communication, education, mindfulness, gradual exposure, and professional support are essential tools in fostering a positive and fulfilling anal play experience. Embracing these challenges as part of the exploration can ultimately lead to greater intimacy, pleasure, and self-acceptance.

Coping with Negative Reactions from Society

In a world that often stigmatizes sexual exploration, particularly anal play, it is essential to develop strategies for coping with negative reactions from society. The journey of embracing one's sexual desires can be met with judgment, misunderstanding, and even hostility. This section aims to provide insights into the theories behind societal reactions, the problems they create, and practical examples of how to navigate these challenges.

Understanding Societal Stigma

Societal stigma surrounding anal play often stems from deeply rooted cultural, religious, and social beliefs about sexuality. Theories of stigma, such as Goffman's *stigma theory*, suggest that individuals who engage in behaviors outside societal norms may be labeled as deviant. This labeling can lead to discrimination, social isolation, and internalized shame.

$$S = f(N, R, C) \tag{33}$$

Where:

- S = Stigma experienced
- N = Norms of society
- R = Reactions from others
- C = Cultural context

The function illustrates that stigma is a function of societal norms, reactions, and cultural context. Understanding this can help individuals contextualize their experiences and reduce feelings of isolation.

Common Negative Reactions

Negative reactions can manifest in various forms, including:

- **Judgmental Attitudes:** Friends, family, or peers may express disapproval or ridicule.

- **Discrimination:** Some may face exclusion from social groups or professional repercussions.

- **Internalized Shame:** Individuals may internalize societal negativity, leading to feelings of guilt or shame about their desires.

These reactions can create significant emotional challenges, impacting self-esteem and mental health.

Coping Strategies

To effectively cope with negative societal reactions, consider the following strategies:

1. Build a Supportive Community   Seek out like-minded individuals who share your interests and values. Online forums, local meetups, and sex-positive groups can provide a safe space for discussion and support. Surrounding yourself with a supportive community can help counteract negative societal messages.

2. Educate Yourself and Others   Knowledge is power. Understanding the anatomy, benefits, and safety of anal play can help you articulate your choices confidently. Sharing this information with others can dispel myths and reduce stigma. For example, discussing the health benefits of anal play, such as improved intimacy and enhanced pleasure, can shift the conversation from judgment to understanding.

3. Practice Self-Compassion   Recognize that your desires are valid and deserving of exploration. Self-compassion involves treating yourself with kindness and understanding, especially when faced with external negativity. Techniques such as mindfulness meditation can help cultivate a more compassionate mindset.

4. Establish Boundaries   It is essential to set boundaries with individuals who are disrespectful or judgmental about your sexual choices. Communicate clearly about what is acceptable in your interactions. For instance, if a friend makes disparaging comments about anal play, express that such remarks are hurtful and not welcome.

5. Seek Professional Support If negative societal reactions lead to significant emotional distress, consider seeking support from a mental health professional. Therapy can provide a safe space to process feelings of shame, anxiety, or depression related to societal stigma.

Real-Life Examples

Consider the story of Jamie, who faced backlash from friends after coming out as an anal enthusiast. Initially, Jamie felt isolated and ashamed. However, by joining an online community of sex-positive individuals, Jamie found support and validation. Through education and open dialogue, Jamie was able to educate friends about the joys and safety of anal play, shifting their perspectives over time.

Another example is Alex, who experienced workplace discrimination after discussing their sexual preferences. Alex chose to establish boundaries with colleagues, refusing to engage in conversations that belittled their desires. By focusing on self-compassion and seeking therapy, Alex was able to reclaim their sense of self-worth and navigate the challenging environment with resilience.

Conclusion

Coping with negative reactions from society is an ongoing process that requires resilience, education, and support. By understanding the roots of societal stigma, employing effective coping strategies, and building a supportive community, individuals can navigate the complexities of their sexual journeys with confidence and pride. Embracing your desires is a powerful act of self-love, and it is essential to remember that you are not alone in this journey. Celebrate your anal journey, and let it empower you to live authentically and unapologetically.

Seeking Professional Help and Support

In the journey of exploring anal pleasure, individuals may encounter various challenges that can affect their experience and enjoyment. These challenges can range from physical discomfort to emotional barriers, and sometimes the stigma surrounding anal play can create feelings of shame or guilt. In such cases, seeking professional help and support can be a valuable step towards overcoming these obstacles and enhancing one's sexual experiences.

Understanding the Need for Support

The necessity for professional support arises when individuals face issues that are beyond their personal coping mechanisms. These issues may include:

- **Physical Discomfort:** Pain during anal play can sometimes signal underlying medical conditions such as anal fissures, hemorrhoids, or other gastrointestinal issues. Consulting a healthcare professional can help identify these conditions and provide appropriate treatment.

- **Emotional Challenges:** Feelings of anxiety, shame, or guilt related to anal play can stem from societal stigma or personal beliefs. A therapist specializing in sexual health can assist individuals in navigating these feelings and fostering a healthier relationship with their sexuality.

- **Relationship Dynamics:** If anal play is causing tension or conflict within a relationship, seeking couples therapy can facilitate open communication and help partners align their desires and boundaries.

Types of Professionals to Consider

When seeking support, individuals may consider various types of professionals, each providing unique perspectives and expertise:

- **Sex Therapists:** These professionals specialize in sexual health and can provide guidance on overcoming emotional barriers, improving communication with partners, and enhancing sexual experiences. They often use evidence-based approaches to address issues such as performance anxiety or sexual dysfunction.

- **Medical Practitioners:** Physicians, especially those specializing in gastroenterology or sexual health, can address any physical concerns related to anal play. They can offer medical advice, treatment options, and referrals to specialists if needed.

- **Counselors and Psychologists:** Mental health professionals can help individuals explore deeper emotional issues, such as trauma or body image concerns, that may affect their sexual experiences. They provide a safe space for discussing feelings and developing coping strategies.

Finding the Right Professional

Finding the right professional can be a crucial step in ensuring a supportive and productive experience. Here are some tips for selecting a suitable therapist or medical practitioner:

- **Research Credentials:** Look for professionals with specific training in sexual health or therapy. Verify their credentials and areas of expertise to ensure they are equipped to address your concerns.

- **Read Reviews:** Online reviews and testimonials can provide insights into other clients' experiences. Look for professionals who have a reputation for being non-judgmental and supportive.

- **Initial Consultation:** Many therapists offer an initial consultation. Use this opportunity to gauge their approach, ask questions about their experience with anal play, and assess your comfort level with them.

- **Discuss Goals:** Be clear about your goals for seeking help. Whether you want to address physical discomfort, enhance pleasure, or navigate emotional barriers, communicating your objectives can help the professional tailor their approach to your needs.

Examples of Situations Requiring Professional Support

Consider the following scenarios that illustrate when seeking professional help may be beneficial:

- **Physical Pain during Anal Play:** An individual experiences consistent pain during anal intercourse, leading to anxiety and avoidance of the activity. A visit to a medical practitioner reveals an anal fissure, which is treated, allowing the individual to enjoy anal play without discomfort.

- **Emotional Barriers:** A couple is interested in exploring anal play but faces ongoing conflict due to one partner's feelings of shame. They seek the assistance of a sex therapist who helps them communicate openly about their desires and fears, ultimately enhancing their intimacy and pleasure.

- **Navigating Relationship Dynamics:** In a polyamorous relationship, one partner feels left out during anal play sessions. They seek couples therapy to address their feelings and establish boundaries that respect everyone's desires, leading to a more harmonious and fulfilling sexual dynamic.

Conclusion

Seeking professional help and support is a proactive step towards enhancing your anal play experiences. Whether addressing physical discomfort, emotional barriers, or relationship dynamics, professionals can provide valuable guidance and resources. Remember, embracing your desires and seeking support is a sign of strength, and it can lead to greater pleasure and fulfillment in your sexual journey.

$$\text{Support} = \text{Understanding} + \text{Communication} + \text{Professional Guidance} \quad (34)$$

By prioritizing your well-being and seeking the right support, you can unlock the full potential of your anal journey, transforming challenges into opportunities for growth and pleasure.

Conclusion

Embracing Your Anal Journey

The journey into anal pleasure is not merely a physical exploration; it is a profound rite of passage that invites you to delve deep into your desires, challenge societal norms, and ultimately embrace your authentic self. This section aims to empower you to navigate your unique anal journey with confidence, joy, and a sense of adventure.

Understanding Your Journey

The first step in embracing your anal journey is to recognize that it is uniquely yours. Each individual's experience with anal play is influenced by personal desires, past experiences, and emotional readiness. The journey can be filled with excitement, curiosity, and sometimes apprehension. It is essential to understand that these feelings are valid and a natural part of the exploration process.

The Importance of Self-Discovery

Anal play can serve as a powerful tool for self-discovery. Engaging with your body in new ways can unlock hidden aspects of your sexuality. Consider the following points:

- **Exploration of Sensation**: Anal play introduces a variety of sensations that can enhance your overall sexual experience. The body is a complex map of pleasure zones, and discovering these can lead to heightened arousal and satisfaction.

- **Breaking Taboos**: Society often stigmatizes anal play, labeling it as taboo or inappropriate. By embracing your anal journey, you challenge these norms, allowing yourself to redefine pleasure on your own terms.

- **Empowerment through Knowledge**: Educating yourself about anal anatomy, techniques, and safety can empower you to take control of your sexual experiences. Knowledge is liberating; it equips you to make informed decisions and communicate effectively with partners.

Navigating Challenges

As with any journey, challenges may arise. It is crucial to approach these hurdles with patience and understanding. Here are some common challenges and strategies to overcome them:

- **Fear of Pain**: Pain is often a significant concern when considering anal play. It is essential to remember that discomfort can be minimized through proper preparation, including relaxation techniques, adequate lubrication, and gradual exploration. Always listen to your body and proceed at a pace that feels comfortable for you.

- **Emotional Barriers**: Past experiences, societal conditioning, or personal insecurities may create emotional barriers to anal play. Journaling, discussing your feelings with trusted friends, or seeking professional guidance can help you process these emotions and move forward.

- **Communication with Partners**: Open dialogue with your partner(s) is vital for a fulfilling anal journey. Establishing trust and discussing desires, boundaries, and safety can enhance intimacy and ensure a positive experience for everyone involved.

Celebrating Milestones

As you progress on your anal journey, it is essential to celebrate your milestones, no matter how small they may seem. Each step forward is an achievement worth acknowledging. Consider keeping a journal to document your experiences, noting the techniques that resonate with you, the sensations you enjoy, and any new discoveries about your body and desires.

Finding Joy in the Process

Embracing your anal journey means finding joy in the exploration itself. Instead of focusing solely on the end goal of pleasure, allow yourself to savor the process of discovery. Engage in playful experimentation, try new techniques, and share laughter and intimacy with your partner(s). Remember that pleasure comes in many forms, and the journey itself can be as fulfilling as the destination.

Continuing the Exploration

Your anal journey does not have to end after a few experiences. Embrace a mindset of continuous exploration. As you become more comfortable with anal play, consider expanding your horizons by exploring different techniques, toys, and scenarios. This could include:

- **Experimenting with Different Toys**: Each toy offers a unique experience. Explore various shapes, sizes, and materials to find what resonates with you.//
- **Incorporating Roleplay**: Roleplay can add an exciting layer to your anal journey, allowing you to explore fantasies and power dynamics in a safe and consensual environment.
- **Engaging in Workshops or Communities**: Seek out workshops, forums, or local communities focused on anal play. Connecting with others who share your interests can provide support, new ideas, and a sense of belonging.

Conclusion: Embracing the Anal Addict Within

Ultimately, embracing your anal journey is about accepting and celebrating your desires without shame. It is an invitation to explore the depths of your pleasure, challenge societal norms, and create a fulfilling sexual life that reflects your true self. As you continue on this path, remember that every person's journey is unique, and there is no right or wrong way to explore. Embrace the anal addict within you, and let your journey be one of joy, exploration, and empowerment.

Celebrating Personal Growth and Exploration

As we journey through the realms of our sexual desires, particularly in the context of anal play, it is essential to recognize and celebrate our personal growth and exploration. This journey is not merely about physical pleasure; it encompasses emotional, psychological, and relational dimensions that contribute to a more profound understanding of ourselves and our desires.

CONCLUSION

The Journey of Self-Discovery

Engaging in anal play often acts as a catalyst for self-discovery. Many individuals find that exploring this taboo area of their sexuality allows them to confront and dismantle internalized beliefs and societal stigmas. As we navigate our desires, we may encounter various emotions, from excitement to fear. Acknowledging these feelings is crucial; it reflects our willingness to embrace our complexities.

> "The only way to deal with fear is to face it head-on. By exploring what we desire, we reclaim our power over our bodies and our pleasure."

Self-discovery can manifest in several ways:

- **Understanding Boundaries:** Through exploration, we learn what feels good and what does not. This understanding is foundational in establishing personal boundaries that enhance our sexual experiences.
- **Embracing Vulnerability:** Anal play often requires a level of vulnerability that can be both daunting and liberating. Embracing this vulnerability can lead to deeper intimacy with ourselves and our partners.
- **Enhancing Communication:** As we explore anal play, we must communicate our desires, limits, and experiences with our partners. This practice not only enriches our sexual encounters but also strengthens our relationships.

The Role of Reflection

Reflection is a powerful tool in celebrating personal growth. After engaging in anal play, taking time to reflect on the experience can yield valuable insights. Consider the following questions:

1. What did I enjoy about the experience?
2. Were there any moments of discomfort, and how did I address them?
3. How did my partner and I communicate during the experience?
4. What have I learned about my desires and boundaries?

Reflecting on these questions can help individuals process their experiences and celebrate their growth. It allows for a deeper understanding of one's sexual identity and can pave the way for further exploration.

Acknowledging Challenges and Triumphs

Personal growth often involves navigating challenges. For many, the journey into anal play can be fraught with fears related to pain, societal judgment, or the fear of not being accepted by partners. Acknowledging these challenges is not a sign of weakness but a testament to the courage it takes to explore one's sexuality.

> "Every challenge faced is a step toward liberation. Each triumph, no matter how small, deserves to be celebrated."

For instance, consider the journey of an individual who initially experienced discomfort during anal play. Through education, communication, and gradual exploration, they learned to relax and enjoy the experience. Celebrating this triumph is essential; it reinforces the idea that growth is a continuous process.

Community and Connection

Another critical aspect of celebrating personal growth is recognizing the importance of community. Engaging with others who share similar interests can provide support, validation, and inspiration. Whether through workshops, online forums, or local meetups, connecting with fellow anal enthusiasts can foster a sense of belonging.

- **Sharing Experiences:** Sharing stories and experiences with others can help normalize anal play and reduce stigma. It can also provide new insights and techniques that enhance personal exploration.

- **Learning from Others:** Engaging with a community allows individuals to learn from the experiences of others. This exchange of knowledge can empower individuals to explore their desires more fully.

The Celebration of Sexual Identity

Ultimately, celebrating personal growth in anal play is about embracing one's sexual identity. Each exploration, each moment of pleasure, and each boundary pushed contributes to a richer understanding of who we are as sexual beings.

> "Your sexual journey is uniquely yours. Celebrate every step, every discovery, and every moment of pleasure."

In conclusion, the journey of personal growth and exploration in anal play is multifaceted. By embracing our desires, reflecting on our experiences, acknowledging challenges, connecting with community, and celebrating our sexual identity, we can unlock a world of extreme pleasure and self-acceptance.

The path may be filled with twists and turns, but every moment spent exploring is a testament to our courage and desire to live authentically. As we continue on this journey, let us celebrate not only the pleasure we discover but also the profound growth that comes from embracing the anal addict within.

Finding Joy in Anal Pleasure

Finding joy in anal pleasure is a journey of self-discovery, empowerment, and connection. It transcends mere physical sensations, delving into emotional and psychological realms that can enhance your overall sexual experience. In this section, we will explore the multifaceted nature of anal pleasure, the importance of a positive mindset, and practical ways to cultivate joy in your anal play.

The Nature of Pleasure

Pleasure is a complex interplay of physical sensations, emotional responses, and psychological states. Anal pleasure specifically engages various nerve endings and erogenous zones, leading to unique experiences that can be both intense and fulfilling. Understanding this interplay can enhance your ability to enjoy anal play.

The human body is equipped with a rich network of nerves, particularly in the anal region. The anal sphincter and surrounding tissues contain a high concentration of nerve endings, making them highly sensitive to touch, pressure, and temperature. Engaging these areas can lead to pleasurable sensations that are often underestimated.

The Psychological Aspect of Pleasure

To truly find joy in anal pleasure, it's crucial to address the psychological barriers that may exist. Many individuals harbor fears or misconceptions about anal play, often rooted in societal stigma. Overcoming these barriers can significantly enhance your enjoyment.

- **Self-acceptance:** Embrace your desires without shame. Acknowledge that seeking pleasure, including anal pleasure, is a natural and healthy aspect of human sexuality.

- **Positive Mindset:** Approach anal play with curiosity and openness. Replace negative thoughts with affirmations that celebrate your body and its capacity for pleasure.

- **Visualization Techniques:** Use visualization to enhance arousal. Imagine the sensations you wish to experience, focusing on the feelings of pleasure and connection.

Creating a Joyful Environment

The environment in which you engage in anal play can significantly impact your experience. Creating a safe, comfortable, and inviting space can enhance your ability to relax and enjoy the moment.

- **Setting the Mood:** Dim the lights, play soft music, and eliminate distractions. A serene environment can heighten your senses and allow you to fully immerse yourself in the experience.

- **Incorporating Rituals:** Develop personal rituals that signal the beginning of your anal play. This could include a warm bath, scented candles, or even a short meditation to center your mind.

- **Using Affirmations:** Before engaging in anal play, recite affirmations that reinforce your confidence and desire. Phrases like "I embrace my body and its pleasures" can help shift your mindset.

Communicating with Your Partner

If you are engaging in anal play with a partner, open communication is essential for mutual enjoyment. Discussing desires, boundaries, and preferences can enhance the experience for both partners.

- **Expressing Desires:** Share what you find pleasurable and what you hope to explore. This could include specific techniques, toys, or sensations you wish to try.

- **Checking In:** During anal play, regularly check in with your partner to ensure they are comfortable and enjoying the experience. Use verbal cues or non-verbal signals to maintain open lines of communication.

- **Aftercare:** After engaging in anal play, take time for aftercare. This can include cuddling, discussing the experience, or simply enjoying each other's presence. Aftercare reinforces intimacy and connection.

Exploring Techniques for Enhanced Pleasure

Finding joy in anal pleasure often involves experimentation with various techniques and methods. Here are some approaches to consider:

- **Breath Control:** Use deep breathing to enhance relaxation and pleasure. Inhale deeply before penetration and exhale slowly during the process to help your body adjust.
- **Gradual Exploration:** Start with gentle touches and gradually increase intensity. This method allows your body to acclimate and can lead to heightened pleasure.
- **Combining Sensations:** Experiment with combining anal play with other forms of stimulation, such as clitoral or penile stimulation. This multi-faceted approach can create more intense and pleasurable experiences.

The Role of Lubrication

Lubrication is a key factor in ensuring comfort and pleasure during anal play. The anal region does not produce natural lubrication, so using an appropriate lubricant is essential.

- **Choosing the Right Lubricant:** Opt for high-quality, body-safe lubricants. Water-based lubricants are versatile, while silicone-based options provide longer-lasting glide.
- **Experimenting with Temperature:** Consider using warming or cooling lubricants to enhance sensations. These can add an exciting element to your anal play.
- **Reapplication:** Don't hesitate to reapply lubricant as needed. Keeping the area well-lubricated is crucial for comfort and enjoyment.

Celebrating Your Experiences

Finally, finding joy in anal pleasure involves celebrating your experiences, regardless of the outcome. Every exploration is an opportunity for growth and self-discovery.

- **Reflecting on Experiences:** After engaging in anal play, take time to reflect on what you enjoyed and what you might want to explore further. Journaling can be a helpful tool for this reflection.

- **Sharing with Your Partner:** Discuss your experiences with your partner, celebrating the moments of connection and pleasure. This reinforces intimacy and can deepen your bond.

- **Embracing Growth:** Understand that pleasure is a journey. Each experience contributes to your understanding of your body and desires, paving the way for future explorations.

Conclusion

Finding joy in anal pleasure is a rewarding journey that encompasses physical sensations, emotional connections, and personal growth. By embracing your desires, cultivating a positive mindset, and fostering open communication, you can unlock new dimensions of pleasure. Remember, the path to joy is unique for everyone—celebrate your journey and the pleasures it brings.

$$\text{Joy in Anal Pleasure} = \text{Self-Acceptance} + \text{Positive Mindset} + \text{Communication} + \text{Exploration} \tag{35}$$

Continuing to Expand Your Sexual Horizons

As you embark on your anal journey, it's crucial to recognize that sexual exploration is an ongoing process. Expanding your sexual horizons involves a commitment to learning, experimenting, and embracing new experiences. This section aims to inspire you to continue your exploration beyond the boundaries of anal play, encouraging you to discover the vast landscape of sexual pleasure.

The Importance of Exploration

Exploration is at the heart of sexual empowerment. It allows you to connect with your body, understand your desires, and discover what truly brings you pleasure. Each experience, whether pleasurable or challenging, contributes to your sexual growth. Embracing this journey means being open to new ideas, techniques, and sensations that may enhance your enjoyment of anal play and sex in general.

Broadening Your Sexual Repertoire

Expanding your sexual horizons can take many forms. Here are some avenues to explore:

- **Diverse Techniques:** As you become more comfortable with anal play, consider incorporating various techniques and styles. For instance, try different types of anal toys, explore new positions, or experiment with temperature play using warmed or cooled items. Each variation can provide a fresh perspective on pleasure.

- **Communication:** Engage in open dialogues with your partner(s) about your desires and fantasies. Sharing your thoughts can lead to discovering mutual interests and new experiences that you may not have considered before. Communication fosters intimacy and trust, essential elements for any sexual exploration.

- **Workshops and Classes:** Attend workshops or classes focused on sexual techniques, including anal play. These environments offer opportunities to learn from experienced educators, ask questions, and practice in a safe space. Knowledge gained in such settings can enhance your confidence and skill level.

- **Reading and Research:** Delve into literature that discusses sexuality, anatomy, and pleasure techniques. Books, articles, and online resources can provide valuable insights and new ideas. Consider exploring topics like BDSM, tantra, or sexual health to enrich your understanding of pleasure.

- **Incorporating Sensation Play:** Sensation play can heighten your anal experiences. Experiment with different textures, pressures, and sensations, such as using feathers, ice, or wax. The interplay of sensations can lead to heightened arousal and deeper connections with your body and partner.

Addressing Challenges and Embracing Growth

As you expand your sexual horizons, you may encounter challenges. These could include fears, insecurities, or societal stigma surrounding certain practices. Addressing these issues is crucial for personal growth. Here are some strategies to help you navigate potential obstacles:

- **Self-Reflection:** Take time to reflect on your feelings and beliefs about your sexual desires. Journaling can be a helpful tool for exploring your thoughts, allowing you to identify areas where you might feel restricted or uncertain.

- **Seek Support:** Surround yourself with supportive individuals who encourage your exploration. This could include friends, partners, or online communities that share similar interests. Engaging with like-minded individuals can provide comfort and affirmation.

- **Therapy and Counseling:** If you find that past experiences or societal pressures hinder your sexual exploration, consider seeking professional help. A therapist specializing in sexual health can provide guidance and support as you navigate your feelings and desires.

The Joy of Discovery

The journey of sexual exploration is not solely about the destination; it's about the joy of discovery. Each new experience, whether it leads to pleasure or discomfort, contributes to your understanding of your body and desires. Celebrate your achievements, no matter how small, and recognize that every step you take is a part of your unique sexual journey.

Embracing Your Inner Anal Addict

As you continue to explore and expand your sexual horizons, embrace the idea of being an "anal addict." This concept transcends mere physical pleasure; it embodies a mindset of curiosity, acceptance, and joy in your sexual experiences. Allow yourself to indulge in your desires without shame or guilt. Remember, your sexual journey is yours to define, and it should be filled with pleasure, exploration, and empowerment.

Conclusion

In conclusion, expanding your sexual horizons is a rewarding and transformative journey. By embracing exploration, broadening your repertoire, addressing challenges, and celebrating your discoveries, you can unlock deeper levels of pleasure and connection. Continue to seek out new experiences, communicate openly with your partners, and cultivate a mindset of curiosity. Your journey is just beginning, and the possibilities for pleasure are limitless.

Embracing the Anal Addict Within

The journey into anal pleasure is not merely a physical exploration; it is a profound journey of self-discovery and acceptance. Embracing the "anal addict" within you means recognizing and celebrating your desires without shame or fear. This section delves into the empowering aspects of accepting your passion for anal play, the psychological benefits it can bring, and how to integrate this part of your identity into your broader sexual experience.

CONCLUSION

Understanding Your Desires

Your desire for anal pleasure is a natural extension of your sexuality. It's essential to understand that this craving is not something to be ashamed of but rather an integral part of your sexual identity. According to Kinsey's research on human sexuality, many individuals experience varying degrees of interest in anal play, highlighting its commonality. Embracing this part of yourself can lead to greater self-acceptance and confidence.

The Psychological Benefits of Acceptance

Accepting your desire for anal play can have significant psychological benefits. It can lead to:

- **Increased Self-Esteem:** Acknowledging and embracing your sexual preferences can enhance your self-image. When you accept who you are, you project confidence, which can be attractive to potential partners.

- **Reduced Anxiety:** Many individuals experience anxiety surrounding their sexual desires. By openly embracing your interest in anal play, you can alleviate feelings of guilt or shame, leading to a more relaxed and enjoyable sexual experience.

- **Enhanced Intimacy:** Sharing your desires with a partner can deepen intimacy. It fosters an environment of trust and openness, allowing both partners to explore their fantasies together.

Integrating Anal Pleasure into Your Sexual Identity

To fully embrace your anal addict identity, consider the following strategies:

1. **Educate Yourself:** Knowledge is power. Read literature, attend workshops, or engage in discussions about anal play. Understanding the anatomy, techniques, and safety precautions can empower you to explore confidently.

2. **Communicate Openly:** Discuss your desires with your partner(s). Use open-ended questions to encourage dialogue about fantasies, boundaries, and interests. For example, you might ask, "How do you feel about exploring anal play together?" This can open the door to deeper conversations about mutual desires.

3. **Experiment and Explore:** Allow yourself to experiment without judgment. Try different techniques, toys, and positions. Keep a journal to document your experiences, feelings, and discoveries. This can help you reflect on your journey and track your growth.

4. **Join a Community:** Seek out communities, both online and offline, where you can share experiences and learn from others. Engaging with fellow anal enthusiasts can provide support and reduce feelings of isolation.

Addressing Societal Stigma

Despite the growing acceptance of diverse sexual practices, societal stigma surrounding anal play persists. It's crucial to confront these societal pressures and recognize that your desires are valid. Here are some strategies to combat stigma:

- **Challenge Negative Beliefs:** Identify and challenge any negative beliefs you may hold about anal play. Replace them with affirmations that celebrate your sexual identity.

- **Educate Others:** Share your knowledge with friends or partners who may hold misconceptions about anal play. Providing accurate information can help dispel myths and promote understanding.

- **Practice Self-Compassion:** Be kind to yourself. Understand that societal pressures can be challenging, and it's okay to feel conflicted. Engage in self-care practices that reinforce your self-worth and acceptance.

Celebrating Your Journey

As you embrace your anal addict identity, take time to celebrate your journey. Reflect on the progress you've made, both in your sexual exploration and personal growth. Consider the following ways to celebrate:

1. **Host a Celebration:** Organize a gathering with friends who share your interests. This can be a space to share experiences, learn from each other, and celebrate your shared passion for anal play.

2. **Create a Ritual:** Develop a personal ritual that honors your journey. This could be as simple as lighting a candle before engaging in anal play or writing a letter to yourself acknowledging your desires and growth.

3. **Share Your Story:** If you feel comfortable, share your experiences through writing, blogging, or speaking. Your story can inspire others to embrace their desires and foster a more accepting environment around anal play.

Conclusion

Embracing the anal addict within is a liberating experience that can lead to profound self-acceptance and joy. By understanding your desires, addressing societal stigma, and integrating anal pleasure into your sexual identity, you can unlock new levels of intimacy and fulfillment. Remember, your journey is uniquely yours—celebrate it, embrace it, and let it empower you to explore the vast landscape of sexual pleasure.

In the words of Betty Dodson, "Your body is a playground, so play!" Allow yourself to explore, enjoy, and embrace every part of your sexual identity, including the thrilling world of anal pleasure. You are not alone in this journey; there is a vibrant community of fellow enthusiasts who celebrate and support your exploration. So, step boldly into your desires, and let the anal addict within you shine brightly.

Index

a, 2–4, 6–9, 11, 12, 14–17, 19–21, 23–28, 31–35, 37–44, 46, 47, 49, 50, 52, 53, 55, 57–60, 62, 65, 66, 68–71, 74, 76–81, 84–86, 88, 90, 93–99, 101–108, 110, 113–116, 118, 121–124, 126, 127, 129, 130, 132–143, 145, 147–162, 164, 167, 169–173, 175–177, 179–185, 187–191, 193–202, 204
ability, 44, 98, 108, 199, 200
acceptance, 2, 3, 6, 8, 189, 199, 204
access, 99, 130, 131, 133
acclimatization, 71
achievement, 195
act, 3, 8, 71, 109, 113, 132, 151, 191
action, 161
activity, 8, 11, 46, 51, 52, 111, 167
adaptation, 153
addict, 196, 199, 204, 205
addition, 64, 70, 139
advance, 61, 151, 160
adventure, 101, 118, 132, 147, 182, 194
advice, 185
aftercare, 47, 53, 110, 149, 151, 172–174
agreement, 8
Alex, 46, 47, 191
ambiguity, 167
amount, 184
anatomy, 14, 16, 19, 21, 23, 24, 26–29, 31, 33, 34, 37, 43, 66, 68, 70, 74, 76, 79, 95, 101, 103, 105, 107, 108, 188, 190
angle, 72, 99
ankle, 130, 133
anticipation, 67, 69, 102, 149
anus, 12, 14, 16, 17, 19, 24, 26, 27, 29, 53, 55, 57, 69, 76, 86, 95, 103, 104, 113, 126, 127, 129, 145
anxiety, 4, 5, 64, 65, 69, 71, 75, 76, 101, 102, 186–189, 191
application, 58, 139
apprehension, 44, 194
approach, 18, 38, 45, 71, 119, 141, 154, 184, 195
area, 14, 15, 19, 21, 24, 27, 46, 55, 60, 68–70, 74, 76, 77, 86, 99, 106, 127, 130, 131, 133, 139, 145, 197
arise, 10, 44, 57, 59, 67, 72, 105,

107, 128, 159, 165, 182, 183, 195
arousal, 19, 25, 27, 31, 37–39, 68–70, 102, 121, 131, 132, 137–140, 142, 147
array, 47
art, 101, 150
aspect, 13, 39, 44, 47, 50, 53, 59, 70, 122, 134, 136, 162, 170, 189, 198
association, 43
assurance, 11
atmosphere, 46, 149
attention, 13, 103
avenue, 33, 95
avoidance, 187
awareness, 73

back, 98
backlash, 191
bacteria, 55
balance, 66, 124
barrier, 4, 5
base, 127
basic, 22
basis, 47
BDSM, 116, 122, 134, 135, 148, 150, 155, 158–160, 162, 167, 170
beauty, 152
bedding, 46
beginning, 204
behavior, 156, 159
being, 12, 46, 50, 72, 73, 152, 172, 194, 198, 202, 204
belly, 37
betrayal, 187
birth, 33
bladder, 31, 60

blanket, 47
blood, 24
bloodstream, 55
blowing, 90, 126
body, 13, 16, 18, 23–26, 28, 37, 39, 54, 60, 65, 68, 70–72, 74, 86, 88, 95, 99, 101, 102, 104, 107, 108, 116, 126, 129, 138, 139, 146, 184, 185, 194, 195, 199, 202, 204
bond, 46, 103, 151, 167, 174
bondage, 129–134, 136–139, 149
bottom, 60
boundary, 51, 164, 198
break, 14
breast, 99
breath, 39
breathing, 39, 70, 104, 129
building, 42, 45–47, 102, 155, 156, 191
bullet, 39
butt, 72, 129, 134

canal, 55, 108
capacity, 39, 150
captive, 149
captor, 149
care, 13, 76, 88, 95, 104, 105, 108, 136, 139, 141, 174, 177
caress, 77
catalyst, 197
cause, 151
caution, 119, 138, 141
cavity, 145
challenge, 1, 157, 175, 179, 194, 196, 198
change, 178
check, 46, 103, 147, 180

Index 211

circulation, 137
clarity, 40, 113
cleaning, 55
cleanliness, 57
clitoris, 38, 39, 74, 99
closeness, 99
cluster, 21
cm, 15
coercion, 9
cold, 145
combat, 70, 157
combination, 42, 98, 118, 125, 134, 148
comfort, 9, 28, 43, 45, 50, 53, 57, 59, 63, 66, 70, 72, 76, 82, 90, 93–95, 101, 102, 104, 121, 126, 128–130, 139, 147, 149, 150, 153, 156, 167, 170, 184, 188, 201
commitment, 46, 47, 62, 136, 162, 177, 202
communication, 3, 8–11, 18, 26, 28, 31, 33, 37, 39, 42, 44, 47, 48, 51, 53, 55, 57, 59, 66, 68, 70–72, 76, 79, 81, 84, 88, 91, 92, 95, 97, 98, 101, 103–105, 108, 110, 112, 113, 115, 116, 118, 123, 124, 126, 129, 131, 132, 134, 136, 139–141, 147, 149–152, 158, 162–167, 169, 170, 172, 175, 177, 180–182, 184, 187, 189, 198, 200
community, 44, 190, 191, 198, 199
compassion, 190, 191
component, 6, 9, 27, 42, 46, 51, 57, 62, 68, 103, 111, 121, 172, 185

composite, 9
concentration, 199
concept, 24, 204
conclusion, 11, 57, 59, 81, 88, 113, 121, 167, 199, 204
conditioning, 185
confidence, 3, 18, 44, 45, 65, 118, 121, 136, 157, 167, 188, 191, 194
connection, 3, 7, 15, 19, 24–26, 28, 39, 47, 50, 73, 90, 98, 99, 101, 113–115, 129, 133, 136, 162, 174, 181, 182, 188, 199, 204
consent, 8–11, 21, 28, 31, 33, 37, 39, 44, 46, 50, 55, 70, 76, 79, 88, 90–92, 95, 97, 105, 113, 115, 118, 123, 124, 132, 134, 136, 139–141, 147, 149, 150, 162, 167, 177, 180, 182
consideration, 82, 106, 177
consistency, 62
contact, 99
context, 44, 63, 121, 134, 135, 139, 150, 152, 177, 189, 196
continue, 18, 73, 174, 196, 199, 202, 204
contrast, 39, 131
control, 26, 43, 44, 54, 60, 99, 113, 122, 127, 128, 132, 136–138, 153, 184
conversation, 156, 164, 190
coordination, 94
core, 132, 175
cornerstone, 9, 40, 110, 162, 164, 170, 175, 177
cost, 107
counselor, 188

couple, 3, 164
courage, 198, 199
courtesy, 170
cowgirl, 99
creativity, 39, 76, 79, 88, 121, 130, 141
culture, 11
curiosity, 42, 194, 204
cycle, 25, 187

damage, 185
dance, 124
day, 46
debriefing, 47, 121, 172
density, 76
depression, 191
deprivation, 138
depth, 99, 104, 113, 115, 184
desensitization, 127
design, 26
desire, 6, 132, 197, 199, 205
destination, 101, 142, 180, 204
detail, 29, 69
dialogue, 2, 3, 9, 11, 48, 51, 53, 110, 113, 156, 164, 170, 177, 191
difference, 82, 185
difficulty, 100
dimension, 69, 116, 121, 132
discipline, 160
discomfort, 3, 13, 47, 52, 69–71, 75, 100–102, 110, 126, 129, 131, 142, 151, 157, 167, 179, 183–185, 191, 194, 198, 204
discovery, 8, 18, 21, 24, 70, 76, 134, 194, 197–199, 201, 204
discrimination, 191

discuss, 11, 46, 47, 52, 59, 121, 150, 177, 179
discussion, 10, 164, 190
distress, 191
doctor, 149
document, 195
Dom, 149
dominance, 105, 113
door, 10, 16
down, 14, 46
duality, 126
dynamic, 39, 118, 122, 129, 134, 149, 151, 158, 159

ease, 104
ecstasy, 126
education, 2, 3, 42, 189, 191, 198
effort, 47, 111, 187
element, 78
embarrassment, 187
empowerment, 3, 8, 21, 152, 189, 196, 199, 202, 204
encounter, 18, 36, 49, 50, 65, 76, 84, 87, 92, 100, 110, 112, 157, 163, 191, 197, 203
end, 16, 26, 196
endurance, 153
engagement, 98
enjoyment, 33, 68, 70, 139, 147, 172, 191, 199, 200, 202
enriching, 143, 149, 182
enthusiasm, 3, 9, 167
enthusiast, 28, 191
environment, 3, 11, 42, 44, 46, 47, 53, 55, 57, 101, 113, 132, 167, 170, 176, 179, 180, 191, 200
equation, 9, 24, 76, 93, 124, 140
equipment, 132, 134, 136

essence, 93, 98
establishment, 51, 156
esteem, 190
examination, 149
example, 38, 39, 151, 190, 191
exchange, 121–123, 136, 139, 148–150
excitement, 44, 46, 90, 101, 132, 133, 186, 194, 197
exercise, 61
exhilaration, 115
experience, 3, 8, 9, 11–13, 15, 19, 21, 23, 25, 28, 32, 35–37, 39–41, 44, 46, 47, 49, 50, 52, 53, 55, 57–59, 63, 65, 69–73, 76, 79–83, 85–90, 92, 93, 95–99, 101–108, 110, 113–116, 118, 121, 126, 129, 131, 132, 134, 136–139, 141, 143, 145, 147–153, 157–160, 162, 167, 170, 172, 174, 177, 180–185, 187–189, 191, 193, 194, 197–200, 202, 204
experiment, 21, 101
experimentation, 201
expertise, 192
exploration, 4, 6, 11, 16, 18, 21, 23, 28, 31, 33, 39, 40, 42–44, 47, 49, 50, 53, 55, 65, 66, 68, 70, 71, 73, 76, 77, 79, 81, 84, 88, 90, 92, 95, 97, 100, 101, 105, 113, 116, 123, 129, 132, 139, 142, 148, 149, 152, 158, 167, 170, 180, 182, 189, 190, 194, 196–199, 201, 202, 204

exposure, 43, 131, 156, 189
expression, 3, 47, 113, 134
expulsion, 26
extension, 19
eye, 99

face, 3, 25, 33, 99, 133, 192, 197
factor, 201
family, 4
fantasy, 39, 147
favorite, 99
fear, 1, 4, 6, 44, 46, 51, 115, 157, 186–188, 197, 198, 204
feature, 72, 184
feedback, 38, 72, 158
feel, 6, 44, 46, 48, 50, 53, 55, 70, 86, 88, 90, 101, 114–116, 121, 132, 147, 150, 167, 174, 175, 180, 184
feeling, 131
fellow, 198
female, 14, 16
finger, 66–69, 72, 74, 76–79, 104, 127, 129
fisting, 103–105, 108–115
flexibility, 63
flogging, 116
floor, 53–55, 60–62
flow, 24
fluid, 31, 34
focus, 39, 68, 70, 126, 150
force, 70
foreplay, 70, 102
form, 8, 60, 160, 167
foundation, 44, 110, 114, 124, 149, 175, 181
framework, 113, 158, 172, 175
freedom, 8, 9, 175
friction, 184

friend, 190
front, 31, 74, 98
fulfillment, 194
fullness, 19, 131
function, 16, 24, 31, 34, 76, 140, 189
functionality, 82, 84
future, 11, 121

gateway, 37, 59
gauge, 147
genital, 24
giver, 113
gland, 27–29, 31, 33, 34, 37, 74
glass, 69
goal, 13, 71, 103, 108, 126, 150, 153
Grafenberg, 74
group, 60
growth, 8, 152, 177, 194, 196–199, 201–203
guidance, 188, 194
guilt, 2, 187, 191, 204

hammock, 60
hand, 103, 104, 113
handle, 35
harm, 151
harmony, 24
head, 197
health, 31, 55, 57, 60, 62, 188, 190, 191
heart, 42, 202
heat, 149, 168
help, 6, 39, 42, 43, 54, 62, 63, 70, 86, 88, 92, 101, 102, 104, 113, 121, 158, 184, 186–191, 193, 194, 197, 203
helplessness, 130
hesitation, 57
high, 12, 53, 104, 184, 187, 199

hold, 131
hook, 138
hooking, 138
hostility, 189
hygiene, 12, 53, 55–57, 107

ice, 131, 149
idea, 198, 204
identity, 197–199, 204, 205
image, 157
impact, 1–3, 98, 99, 116–121, 200
implement, 168
implementation, 159
importance, 6, 8, 10, 11, 33, 40, 43–45, 50, 71, 105, 108, 110, 135, 140, 163, 165–167, 170–172, 177, 198, 199
improvement, 11, 62, 158
in, 1–4, 6, 8–11, 14–16, 19–21, 24, 25, 27, 28, 30, 31, 34, 37, 38, 40, 43, 44, 46–48, 50–53, 55, 56, 60, 62, 63, 66, 68–70, 72–74, 76–79, 81, 82, 90, 93, 94, 98, 99, 101–110, 112–116, 118, 121–124, 126, 129–136, 138–140, 145–152, 155–157, 160–162, 165–168, 170, 172–177, 179–191, 193, 194, 196–202, 204
incorporation, 93
increase, 24, 39, 63, 70, 102, 104, 138, 153, 184
individual, 19, 50, 93, 159, 185, 194, 198
information, 5, 190
injury, 106, 126, 132, 185

insertion, 68, 71–73, 77, 82, 103, 113
insight, 40, 62
inspiration, 198
instance, 3, 8, 39, 43, 134, 157, 190, 198
integration, 118
intensity, 69, 150, 160, 188
interconnectedness, 37
intercourse, 31
interest, 6, 44
interplay, 15, 39, 113, 118, 199
intersection, 124, 126, 129, 132
intimacy, 3, 8, 25, 26, 37, 40, 44, 46, 47, 50, 53, 57, 68, 73, 76, 95, 97–99, 101, 103, 118, 121–123, 126, 129, 134, 137, 139, 141, 142, 149, 152, 158, 167, 172, 174, 180, 185, 187, 189, 190
introduction, 79, 126
invitation, 196
involvement, 9
isolation, 2, 189

Jamie, 191
jealousy, 179
Jessica, 44, 46, 47
journal, 62, 195
journey, 3, 6, 8, 11, 18, 21, 24, 25, 28, 32, 33, 37, 39, 40, 42, 47, 50, 53, 55, 57, 62, 65, 68, 70, 76, 79, 81, 88, 95, 98, 101, 105, 113, 115, 121, 123, 124, 126, 129, 134, 139, 142, 145, 147, 149, 150, 152, 158, 174, 177, 180, 182, 189, 191, 194–196, 198, 199, 202, 204
joy, 65, 68, 113, 118, 194, 196, 199, 201, 204
judgment, 4, 6, 44, 49, 51, 187, 189, 190, 198

Kegel, 61, 62
key, 11, 14, 16, 17, 21, 27, 37, 39, 50, 53, 55, 59, 68, 70, 71, 79, 90, 94, 97, 102, 106, 110, 113, 116, 118, 124, 129, 132, 134, 136, 139, 145, 147, 149, 153, 156, 162, 167, 170, 177, 181, 182, 201
kindness, 190
kissing, 99
knowledge, 4, 18, 28, 76

lack, 4, 5
landscape, 50, 175, 202
lap, 99
lead, 5, 6, 8, 21, 24, 27, 28, 31, 33, 34, 37, 38, 47, 55, 60, 68, 71, 73, 74, 81, 101, 102, 107, 123, 124, 126, 131, 132, 137, 146, 149, 152, 171, 177, 183, 185, 189, 191, 194, 199, 205
level, 43, 104, 114, 129, 149, 187
liberation, 198
lie, 76, 98, 99, 115
life, 196
lifestyle, 180
light, 46, 77, 99
lighting, 46
likelihood, 184
limit, 136

listening, 108
location, 19
loop, 38
lotion, 121
love, 191
lubricant, 12, 43, 53, 58, 69, 72, 129, 184, 201
lubrication, 12, 43, 53, 55, 57, 59, 75, 107, 129, 201

making, 14, 18, 25, 31, 39, 40, 53, 57, 63, 66, 68, 76, 88, 99, 102, 104, 113, 127, 134, 199
male, 26–29, 31, 33, 37
maneuverability, 35
manner, 116, 162, 177
massage, 45, 46, 86, 129
massager, 39
massaging, 69, 70
material, 82
matter, 195, 198, 204
means, 24, 31, 49, 71, 159, 202, 204
mechanism, 164
meditation, 190
method, 167
Michael, 44
mind, 65, 79, 90, 106, 126, 146, 155
mindfulness, 62, 71, 73, 147, 188–190
mindset, 71, 190, 196, 199, 204
miscommunication, 100
misunderstanding, 1, 5, 189
mix, 180
moment, 73, 101, 168, 198–200
motion, 69, 77, 78
movement, 136
muscle, 53
music, 46

myriad, 3, 18, 79, 182

nature, 11, 44, 50, 159, 180, 199
necessity, 57, 192
need, 150, 167
negativity, 190
negotiation, 162, 164
nerve, 14, 15, 19, 21, 24, 31, 68, 74, 76, 127, 139, 145, 199
nervousness, 46
net, 11
network, 19, 68, 74, 199
newfound, 3, 44
nipple, 103
non, 169, 170, 177, 179, 180
novice, 28
nurturing, 172, 174

object, 69, 102
oil, 58
on, 5, 14, 15, 21, 33, 39, 45, 68–70, 72–74, 78, 88, 93, 98, 99, 102, 104, 113, 124, 126, 129, 136, 149, 150, 152, 153, 158, 159, 177, 182, 191, 195–197, 199, 202
one, 18, 24, 39, 40, 59, 70–72, 102–104, 122, 127, 129, 132, 149, 169, 172, 182, 189, 191, 196–198
opening, 16, 26, 67, 74, 76, 77
openness, 164
opportunity, 19, 97, 201
organ, 31, 37
orgasm, 27, 31, 36, 39, 68
other, 3, 13, 24, 28, 32, 37–39, 44, 46, 52, 70, 98, 99, 103, 131, 136, 138, 147, 149, 162, 172, 180

out, 73, 77, 190, 191, 204
outcome, 201
outside, 68, 121
overview, 134

pace, 43, 102, 113, 127
pain, 13, 43, 46, 71, 101, 115, 124–126, 139, 183, 185, 187, 198
part, 6, 27, 47, 49, 52, 55, 68, 74, 185, 189, 194, 204
participant, 3, 170
partner, 13, 25, 28, 35, 38, 39, 43, 44, 46–48, 50, 57, 59, 66, 68–73, 77, 79, 81, 84, 88–93, 98, 99, 102, 104, 105, 108, 114, 121, 122, 127, 129–134, 137–139, 149, 151, 169, 177–179, 184, 200
passage, 194
passion, 204
past, 42, 44, 170, 194
path, 196, 199
pathway, 66
patience, 21, 71, 104, 108, 158, 195
patient, 149
pelvis, 60
penetration, 15, 19, 31, 43, 46, 70, 77, 93–95, 97–99, 101–103, 113, 126–129, 145, 184
penis, 36, 38
perineum, 14, 24, 27, 29, 69, 70
person, 6, 18, 19, 21, 24, 129, 196
perspective, 44
perversion, 4
phenomenon, 24, 31
philosophy, 132

picture, 84
place, 134, 179
plan, 44
play, 1–4, 6, 8–16, 18–21, 25, 26, 28–31, 33, 37, 39–47, 49–57, 59, 60, 62–66, 68–73, 76, 77, 79–81, 85–92, 98, 99, 101, 104–107, 113, 116–122, 124, 126, 128–132, 134–139, 141–150, 152, 153, 155–158, 162–168, 170, 172, 174–177, 179–191, 194, 196–202, 204, 205
playing, 157
pleasure, 1, 3–5, 8, 11, 13–16, 18, 21–29, 31–34, 37–39, 42, 47, 50, 53, 57, 59, 60, 62, 65, 66, 68–71, 74, 76, 77, 79–82, 84, 85, 88, 90–93, 95, 97–101, 103, 105–107, 109, 113, 115, 116, 118, 121, 123–127, 129, 131–134, 139, 141, 142, 145, 147–150, 152, 153, 157, 158, 162, 169, 170, 172, 175, 177, 180–182, 186, 189–191, 194, 196–199, 201, 202, 204
plenty, 43
plug, 129, 134
point, 39, 68, 70
polyamory, 175, 182
position, 87, 93, 95, 98–100, 133, 137, 138
positioning, 98
post, 46, 52

potential, 9, 11, 21, 25, 26, 31, 33, 37, 39, 74, 88, 95, 97, 105, 113, 115, 118, 119, 121, 123, 126, 142, 143, 148, 149, 159, 164, 172, 194, 203
power, 43, 47, 59, 95, 105, 113–116, 121–123, 134, 136, 139, 148–150, 190, 197
practice, 39, 95, 103, 113, 121, 124, 127, 132, 134–136, 139, 150, 172, 174, 185
practitioner, 193
preparation, 42, 43, 53, 55, 63, 65, 66, 68, 71, 88, 103, 108, 150
pressure, 10, 27, 31, 39, 67, 69, 70, 77, 104, 146, 147, 199
pride, 191
principle, 153, 175
priority, 81, 83
process, 2, 11, 46, 47, 53, 72, 73, 104, 113, 151, 152, 181, 191, 194, 197, 198, 202
professional, 185, 189, 191–194
progress, 62, 195
progression, 152
prostate, 27–39, 74–76, 78, 99
proximity, 15, 19, 24, 31

quality, 12, 53, 184
quest, 98
question, 10

range, 44, 47, 101, 139, 142, 145, 157, 171, 184, 186, 191
readiness, 65, 71, 124, 194
realization, 3

realm, 3, 8, 88, 98, 155, 159, 165, 170, 172, 180
reassurance, 121
receiver, 113, 114
receiving, 72, 98, 99, 102, 104, 127, 129
rectum, 17, 29, 31, 33, 37, 55, 74, 76, 108
reflection, 6, 40, 42, 48, 62, 158
region, 14, 17, 18, 21, 24, 199, 201
rejection, 6, 44
relationship, 40, 44, 105, 140, 159, 162, 164, 177, 179, 194
relax, 39, 67, 72, 102, 104, 146, 198, 200
relaxation, 43, 53–55, 63–65, 70, 100, 129, 184
relief, 44
repertoire, 95, 139, 204
report, 25
reputation, 20
resilience, 191
respect, 46, 47, 50, 118, 136, 149–151, 162, 167, 170, 171, 177, 180
response, 37
restraint, 129, 131, 132, 136
result, 2
rhythm, 39, 70, 100
right, 58, 74, 79, 81, 82, 84, 88, 90, 93, 95, 98, 100, 101, 185, 193, 194, 196
ring, 76
risk, 110, 126
rite, 194
role, 4, 14, 20, 21, 31, 34, 39, 72, 76, 106, 134, 147, 149, 150, 157

Index

roleplay, 39, 47, 95, 121–123, 148, 149
rotation, 78
routine, 62, 63, 154
rule, 71

safety, 9, 11, 18, 28, 31, 33, 57, 59, 66, 71, 74, 76, 79, 81–85, 88, 90, 92, 95, 103, 105–107, 116, 118, 123, 126, 127, 132, 134–136, 139, 147, 149, 150, 152, 155, 162, 164, 167, 177, 178, 188, 190, 191
Sarah, 43
satisfaction, 8, 15, 26, 28, 33, 39, 73, 79, 85, 88, 97, 98
scenario, 6, 129, 140, 149, 164
scissor, 78
scrotum, 27, 29
second, 102
section, 3, 6, 8, 11, 14, 26, 29, 33, 37, 40, 44, 47, 50, 53, 55, 57, 63, 66, 68, 71, 74, 76, 79, 82, 85, 88, 90, 98, 105, 108, 110, 113, 116, 118, 121, 124, 126, 129, 132, 134, 136, 139, 142, 145, 148, 150, 155, 159, 162, 164, 167, 170, 172, 175, 177, 183, 185, 189, 194, 199, 202, 204
security, 99
self, 2, 3, 6, 8, 40, 42, 48, 53, 157, 189–191, 194, 196, 197, 199, 201, 204
sensation, 24, 69, 72, 78, 106, 116, 127, 131, 138–147, 149

sense, 8, 9, 25, 73, 99, 121, 122, 130, 132, 191, 194, 198
sensitivity, 15, 19, 24, 31, 70, 77, 139, 145
series, 157
session, 13, 121, 149, 158
set, 180, 190
setting, 51, 167
sex, 3, 6, 39, 116–118, 121–123, 190, 191, 202
sexuality, 1, 4, 6, 49, 126, 175, 194, 197, 198
shame, 1, 2, 4, 6, 49, 187, 189, 191, 196, 204
shape, 35, 82, 84
sharing, 81
shift, 19, 121, 190
side, 100, 104
sight, 138
sign, 194, 198
signal, 88, 102, 150, 184, 185
significance, 164
silence, 46
silicone, 58, 184
silk, 69
situation, 13, 179
size, 19, 82, 84, 150, 184
skill, 156, 158
skin, 69, 77, 130, 145
slate, 57
slave, 155, 156, 158
slavery, 150–152
snugness, 137
society, 3, 4, 189, 191
solo, 33, 66, 70, 79, 81, 85, 87, 88, 91, 129
sound, 138
source, 71, 183
space, 25, 46, 65, 149, 190, 191, 200

spanking, 99, 116, 119–121, 149
specific, 98, 134, 151, 159, 180
spectrum, 24, 93, 113
speed, 70
sperm, 31, 34
sphincter, 26, 67, 72, 76, 104, 108, 127, 153, 199
spot, 15, 19–23, 31, 33, 37, 74–76, 78
stage, 164
start, 43, 46, 48, 82, 101, 129
starting, 68, 70
state, 65
step, 3, 6, 45, 48, 90, 121, 183, 191, 193–195, 198, 204
stigma, 1–4, 40, 42, 44, 157, 189–191, 199, 203
stimulation, 15, 19, 21, 23–25, 27, 28, 32–39, 43, 45, 46, 66–70, 74–78, 85, 86, 93, 98, 99, 103, 129, 130, 132, 134
stop, 13, 51, 75, 102, 131, 150, 167, 185
story, 191
strength, 61, 113, 153, 194
stretch, 108
stretching, 53–55, 63–65
structure, 21, 175
student, 149
style, 99
submission, 105, 113, 149
submissive, 122, 130, 151, 155, 157, 158
success, 177
suggestion, 57
sum, 93
summary, 16, 28
supply, 24

support, 8, 180, 188–192, 194, 198
surrender, 115, 132
symphony, 37
synergy, 70
system, 24

t, 59
taboo, 4, 47, 121, 197
talk, 103
tapestry, 148
teacher, 149
teasing, 68, 145
technique, 67, 68, 76–78, 103, 105, 126, 129, 131, 138
temperature, 69, 145, 147, 149, 199
tension, 54, 63, 75, 104, 184
terrain, 50
testament, 26, 198, 199
texture, 147
theory, 37, 76, 118, 139, 153, 159, 162, 173
therapist, 188, 193
therapy, 191
thought, 19
thrill, 136, 149
thrusting, 15
time, 7, 11, 13, 45, 46, 57, 71, 98, 102, 103, 105, 107, 111, 127, 129, 150, 153, 172, 178, 191, 197
tissue, 19, 21, 74
tool, 127, 151, 155, 180, 194, 197
torture, 139–141
touch, 14, 31, 68, 76, 127, 138, 185, 199
toy, 38, 69, 81, 85, 86, 92, 99, 129, 134
tract, 16, 26
trainee, 150–152

Index

trainer, 150, 152, 157
training, 150–155, 184
transfer, 122
transparency, 167, 179
trauma, 44, 187
treasure, 33
treatment, 185
triumph, 198
trust, 3, 9, 25, 40, 42, 44, 45, 47, 48, 53, 57, 66, 101, 103–105, 110–116, 122–124, 129, 132, 137, 148–152, 155, 158, 162, 167, 170, 172, 175, 177–182, 185, 187, 189
twist, 78
type, 58, 69

understanding, 3, 6, 11, 16, 18, 23, 26, 33, 37, 39, 47, 50, 55, 57, 59, 66, 68, 70, 76, 79, 83, 88, 95, 97, 101, 103, 105, 108, 118, 121, 126, 132, 134, 136, 139, 141, 149, 152, 158, 180, 182, 186, 189–191, 195–198, 204
up, 44, 56, 68, 104
urethra, 19
urgency, 19
use, 12, 38, 39, 43, 53, 57, 72, 76, 88, 93, 127, 129, 136, 138, 139, 146, 149
uterus, 60

vagina, 14, 15, 24, 74, 95
validation, 191, 198

variety, 16, 17, 55, 88, 149, 185
versatility, 130
vibration, 147
vibrator, 39, 69
vice, 24
vulnerability, 111, 114, 115, 131–133, 149, 151, 174

wall, 15, 31, 33, 74
walnut, 31, 33, 37, 74
warming, 68, 69
warmth, 99
water, 58
way, 105, 123, 130, 158, 167, 180, 196, 197
weakness, 198
wealth, 28
weight, 153
well, 43, 46, 50, 61, 68, 70, 121, 127, 136, 152, 194
will, 8, 11, 14, 26, 29, 37, 47, 50, 53, 55, 57, 63, 68, 69, 71, 74, 79, 82, 85, 88, 90, 105, 108, 113, 118, 121, 126, 129, 132, 134, 136, 145, 155, 162, 164, 167, 172, 175, 180, 199
willingness, 21, 37, 50, 70, 101, 182, 197
word, 3, 70, 88, 94, 102, 150, 184
workshop, 3
world, 3, 50, 79, 90, 101, 118, 126, 134, 147, 189, 199
worth, 191, 195
wrist, 130, 133

yourself, 6, 8, 28, 36, 88, 190, 204